BARNES & NOBLE BASICS

getting in
Shape

by Carol Leonetti Dannhauser and
Sandra Michaelson Warren

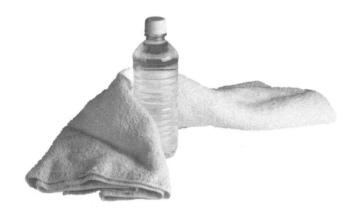

Formerly published as
I need to get in Shape, Now What?!

**BARNES
& NOBLE**
B O O K S

Copyright © 2003 by Silver Lining Books,
an imprint of Barnes & Noble, Inc.

ISBN 0760740259

Originally published in 2000 as *I need to get in Shape,
Now What?!*
Printed and bound in the United States of America.

For information, contact:
Silver Lining Books
122 Fifth Avenue
New York, NY 10011
212-633-4000

Other titles in the **Barnes & Noble Basics**™ series:
Barnes & Noble Basics *Using Your PC*
Barnes & Noble Basics *Wine*
Barnes & Noble Basics *In the Kitchen*
Barnes & Noble Basics *Getting a Job*
Barnes & Noble Basics *Saving Money*
Barnes & Noble Basics *Using the Internet*
Barnes & Noble Basics *Retiring*
Barnes & Noble Basics *Using Your Digital Camera*
Barnes & Noble Basics *Getting Married*
Barnes & Noble Basics *Grilling*
Barnes & Noble Basics *Giving a Presentation*
Barnes & Noble Basics *Buying a House*
Barnes & Noble Basics *Volunteering*
Barnes & Noble Basics *Getting a Grant*
Barnes & Noble Basics *Getting into College*
Barnes & Noble Basics *Golf*

introduction

SONNY CLARK WAS ADAMANT: "I'm going to get in shape if it kills me!!!" She put down her diet soda and sighed. "I just wish I knew how. It's so confusing: one day it's eat pineapple to lose weight, the next it's drink green tea and jump rope, or take vitamin this and that. All I want to do is lose a few pounds and not feel so, well, out of it." Precisely. It's what we all want. The problem is finding a sensible way to go about it. That's where *Barnes & Noble Basics Getting in Shape* comes in. It is full of useful, easy-to-follow information and tips that will both inform and inspire. Want to learn how to actually enjoy exercising? Turn to pages 160–161. Want to know how to tone a particular muscle group? See pages 142–153. Want to see how easy it is to cook healthy meals? Take a look at pages 74–75. It's all here. Consider this book your own personal trainer. Now turn the page and see just how easy and fun it is to get in shape.

Barb Chintz
Editorial Director, the **Barnes & Noble Basics**™ Series

contents

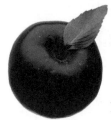

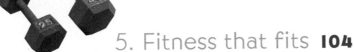

shaping up

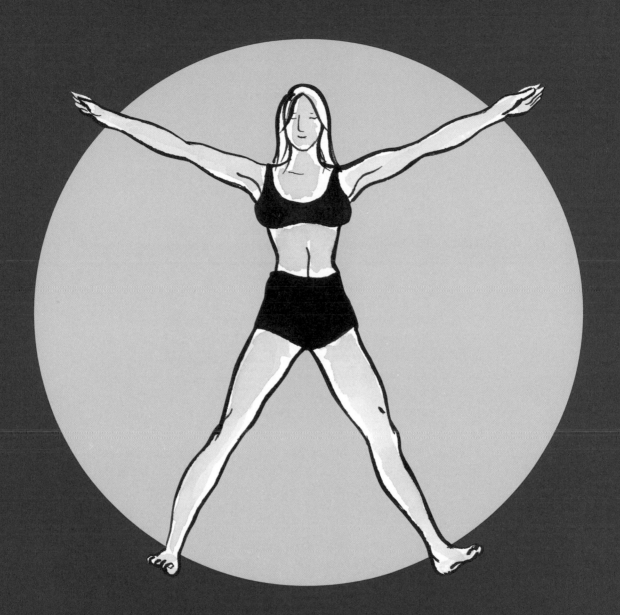

Getting in shape will make you look and feel better. Start smart by evaluating your fitness level right now; then set realistic goals, and devise a plan to attain them.

getting started

You already have

Sometimes, the hardest part about getting in shape—
or doing anything that feels daunting—is getting started. But once
you take a tiny first step, the next step seems easier. Before you
know it, you're on your way!

You already have taken a giant step toward shaping up by reading
this book. Now you need to make healthy eating and exercise a
priority. You *can* do it.

First off, design a program that fits your needs. You wouldn't build
a house without an architectural plan, would you? Same goes for
designing a sound nutrition and fitness strategy. Formulating a plan
takes some work but the payoff lasts a lifetime.

To start building your shape-up program, you need to:
- set your goals
- assess your current weight and fitness level
- understand why you're not in shape now
- psych yourself up
- find realistic ways to add fitness into your daily life

The sections in this chapter will walk you through the entire
process. You can do things right now to get started, but the path
to fitness takes time. Anyone who promises a quick fix is not being
honest. Be patient. If you try to rush it, expecting to accomplish
too much before your body and mind are ready, you might get hurt
or discouraged, and quit. Don't give up before you have the chance
to see and *feel* the results of your efforts. Remember the benefits
and stay focused on your goals.

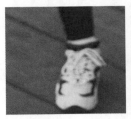
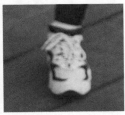

ASK THE EXPERTS

I've never worked out before. Do I have to see a doctor first?
If you're 35 or younger and you're in good health, you probably
are safe adding some exercise to your routine. However, it's
always a wise idea to seek your doctor's advice before beginning
any fitness or weight-loss plan. The President's Council on
Physical Fitness and Sports recommends seeing your doctor
before beginning a shape-up program if you have ever had high
blood pressure; heart problems; strokes; dizziness; breathless-
ness; arthritis; bone or joint problems; problems with your muscles, ligaments, or tendons; other medical conditions such as
back or neck problems; or if you are obese.

I have a bad knee. Does this mean I can't get in shape?
Not at all. Bad knee or not, you can certainly follow the path to
healthful eating. (You'll get all the details in *Nutrition basics*,
Weighing in, and *Eating right*.) As for exercise, there's a great
deal you can do without taxing your knee. Check with your
doctor before starting.

EASE INTO IT

**Don't know where to
start?** Slip on your
sneakers and head
for the mall—before
the stores open.
Many malls open
their doors to walk-
ers each morning.
(The regulars can
tell you how many
times you have to
pass the escalator to
walk a mile.)

setting your goals

Why do you want to get in shape, anyway? So you can zip up those jeans that are languishing in the closet? Lower your cholesterol? Boost your self-esteem? Pump like Arnold? Play tag with your kids? Keep osteoporosis at bay? Beat your college roommate in tennis? Shed a few, or a few dozen, pounds? Limber up those creaky joints? Run a marathon? *Simply feel great?*

Or, you may have fallen off the fitness bandwagon and want a little pick-me-up to regain muscle strength and tone your body. That's okay, too. You want to feel—and look—your best.

Having a goal (like lowering your cholesterol or toning muscles) will be key to your success. Setting a goal, even a small one, will make it easier to stick to a fitness program.

When you put your goals on paper, make sure you're not scowling. There's no way you're going to strive for a goal that doesn't appeal to you. Don't pledge to run three miles a day, for example, if you *hate* to run. Instead, choose an option that sounds fun, like dancing, brisk walking, a step class, or swimming. (You'll learn about all kinds of fun possibilities in *Exercising your options*.) Your goals should encourage, not intimidate, you.

Determine which goals *you* want to accomplish—not what your mate, your mother, or the media wants of you. If you really don't want to make a change, then change won't happen. Remind yourself of the benefits of shaping up. These are the greatest motivators!

Next, figure out which of the goals are realistic. (Given enough time, perhaps they all are!) If you pledge to look like a model or to run a marathon in two months' time, you're probably setting yourself up to fail. Don't try for too much, too soon. If you vow to exercise for an hour each day and you miss a few days, you risk getting discouraged and quitting.

1/1/2001: New Year's resolution. Got to lose 10 pounds.
1/2/2001: Big fight with Hank; ate a pint of ice cream.
Goal: Lose ten pounds.
Method: Stop eating junk food—especially when I'm
upset. Instead, when stress hits, I'll grab an apple, listen
to some music, call a friend, or go for a power walk.

1/3/2001: Went to the zoo with the kids and came
home really tired. Don't like that.
Goal: To feel more energetic.
Method: Walk around the block at least twice a week.

1/6/2001: Party at Joanne's. I get nervous at parties
and usually drink one too many. Then I eat everything
in sight.
Goal: Don't drink more than one alcoholic beverage.
Method: Stay calm and enlist a friend to keep me
company when I start to lose control.

EASE INTO IT

Write your goals in a notebook that you will devote to shaping up. You can be vague. In fact, this might improve your chances of success.

being in shape

Fitness defined

Here's the good news: Because you're reading this book, you must want to get in shape. Or at least be intrigued by the idea. This desire puts you in the fast lane to fitness, well ahead of couch-worshipping, out-of-shape friends and family.

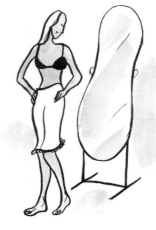

Here's the bad news: Since you're reading this book, you're probably not in shape now. Your muscles might be weak. Your heart and lungs aren't working as efficiently as they could. You might get winded after a flight or two of stairs and have trouble carrying the groceries. You may not eat right, leaving you feeling sluggish.

But not for long. Once you're in shape, the benefits will envelop you like a warm blanket. Here are the four factors to fitness:

- **Cardiorespiratory fitness.** When you're in shape, your heart and lungs operate like a well-oiled engine, delivering oxygen and nutrients where they're needed while removing waste.

- **Muscle strength** and **muscle endurance.** When you're in shape, muscles can exert and sustain force and recover with ease.

- **Flexibility.** This is how well you can move joints and muscles through their natural range of motion. After you shape up, you can sit on the floor in front of the TV, legs outstretched, and reach for the remote near your feet. No pops, pings, or pulls.

- **Body composition.** This tells you how much of your body is fat and how much is not. When you're in shape, the rolls, jiggles, and layers melt away, leaving you lean, fit, and strong.

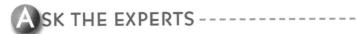

ASK THE EXPERTS

Why do I need to get in shape anyway?

Your health is reason number one. Being in shape reduces the risk of heart disease and osteoporosis. It lowers your cholesterol levels and blood pressure. It reduces the likelihood of certain types of cancer and diabetes. It's the key to a healthy, active life as you age. Then, there's the way you *feel*. Shaping up will improve your quality of life immediately. When you exercise and eat right, you feel wonderful. You look terrific. You move with a spring in your step. Before you know it, you're toned, strong, and able.

Why does getting in shape make me feel better?

In a word: Chemistry. When you exercise, your body releases endorphins—hormones that make you feel good all over. As a result, your stress level shrinks along with the inches on your waistline. You sleep without fits and starts. Exercising also kick-starts your metabolism. Even sitting around doing nothing, a fit body burns more calories than an unfit one. Then there's self-esteem. Once you shape up, you look in the mirror and see firm where there was flab. You're confident and in control. You're happy with your body. Well, *happier*.

fitness quiz

Test your ticker, measure your mass, and factor your fat

What kind of shape are you in now? In order to answer that question, you need to examine a few things: your body composition, waist size, flexibility, muscle strength and endurance, and aerobic (or cardiorespiratory) fitness. Relax. Take a few deep breaths and remember that testing your fitness is simply a tool to help understand where you are and where you want to go. Think of your fitness findings as a road map. You're here and you want to get there. Then figure out the best route.

What will you need? A trusty calculator, tape measure, watch with a second hand, a scale, and, of course, your fitness notebook.

Your Heart Rate. First measure your aerobic fitness, which reflects how well your body transports oxygen and nutrients. Your heart rate is a key indicator of aerobic fitness. To measure your heart rate, take your pulse. (Don't do anything vigorous before the test and try not to smoke or have any caffeine for at least a couple of hours beforehand.) Find a clock with a second hand. Then take your index or middle finger and press lightly on your other wrist, below the base of your thumb. (Feel around—your pulse is there.) If you can't locate it, put your fingers at the outside corner of your eye, then slide them straight down to the carotid artery on your neck. Once you find your pulse, count the beats for 30 seconds. Multiply that by two to get your one-minute **resting heart rate.**

Time to measure your heart rate after a little workout. Go to the local track, hop on a treadmill, or mark out a mile with your car. Before you start the course, walk slowly for about five minutes to warm up. Then, at the beginning of the mile course, note the time

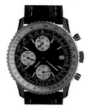 to the second and try to walk or run the mile—or as much of it as you can—as quickly as you can. The second you finish, note the time and immediately measure your pulse. Write down your heart rate and the time.

Your heart rate during exertion is a meaningful gauge you'll return to again and again. First, figure your maximum heart rate. Subtract your age from 220. For example, if you're 35, your maximum heart rate is 185.

Now you want to find your healthy zone, which is 50 to 75 percent of your maximum rate. To find the low end of your range, multiply your maximum rate by 0.50. If you're 35, this would be 185 times 0.50, or 92.5. To get the high end of your range, multiply your maximum by 0.75, which would be 138 for a person who's 35. So, the ideal exertion zone of a 35-year-old ranges from 93 to 140 beats a minute.

When you start shaping up, aim to exercise at the low end of the range and progress toward the high end. The rate you aim for is commonly referred to as your **target heart rate**. If your heart rate exceeds your zone, decrease your exercise intensity (walk or run a little more slowly, for example). If your heart rate is below your zone, try to pick up the pace a bit. As you get in better shape, your heart will begin to pump more efficiently, resulting in fewer pumps (and less wear and tear) to move the same amount of blood.

Test yourself again in six weeks or so and then every couple of months after. Good news: Within six months of a regular exercise program, your resting pulse will probably drop about 10 to 15 beats a minute and you'll run or walk faster, shrinking your time in the mile run or walk.

Your Strength. Muscle strength refers to how much you can lift, push, or pull at one time. But unless you're already in shape, it isn't a good idea to max out: You risk hurting yourself. When you're just getting started, fitness trainers are more apt to test muscle endurance, which marks how well your particular muscle groups hold up under repetitive exercises, such as push-ups, pull-ups, and sit-ups.

EASE INTO IT

Remember, if you have heart problems, high blood pressure, diabetes, bone or joint problems, chest pains, dizziness, breathing problems, or any other medical condition, check with your doctor before beginning any fitness program.

fitness quiz *(cont'd.)*

To measure your upper-body endurance, stretch out on the floor, tummy-side down, and get in a push-up position: Hands below your shoulders and either knees (if you're a woman) or toes (if you're a man) on the floor. Try to push yourself up while maintaining a straight line from your neck to your knees or feet. Can you do it? Can you do five in a row? How about 10? Record the number you can do without resting or compromising your form (and don't hold your breath!). Exhale as you push up.

Next, it's crunch time: testing your abdominal muscles. (Don't do this if you have a bad back.) Lie on your back with your arms crossing your chest. Bend your knees and keep your feet on the floor. Now, try to curl yourself up and lift your shoulder blades off the floor without using momentum. Can you do it? How many can you do correctly without stopping?

Your Flexibility. How flexible are you? How supple are your joints? Flexibility is tricky to measure, as your range of motion might vary greatly from one joint to the next. Flexibility means more than being able to bend or to sit and touch your toes. It ensures balance, agility, and coordination. How flexible you are helps prevent you from falling or injuring yourself when you slip on the ice.

	HEART RATE	
AGE	**TARGET HR ZONE** **50-75 % AVERAGE**	**MAXIMUM HEART RATE** **100 %**
25 years	98-146 beats per minute	195
30 years	95-142 beats per minute	190
35 years	93-138 beats per minute	185
40 years	90-135 beats per minute	180
45 years	88-131 beats per minute	175
50 years	85-127 beats per minute	170

Here's a quick flexibility test:

Walk around for a couple of minutes. Once you feel loose, stand up straight, then bend at the waist. Stretch your fingers toward the floor. Can you touch it? If not, can you touch your toes? (Don't force anything here.) If you don't want to try touching your toes, put a yardstick on the floor and tape across the 15-inch mark. Now, sit on the floor, legs straddling the yardstick, with your torso toward the zero-inch end and your feet 12 inches apart. Line up your heels with the 15-inch tape line. Exhale, and, placing one hand over the other with tips of middle fingers aligned, reach forward as far as you can without bouncing or jerking. Note how far down the yardstick you can reach. (Stop if anything starts to feel uncomfortable.) Can you pass your knees? Can you reach your toes? Do it three times and note your best score.

Now, check how flexible your shoulders are (otherwise known as the "Honey, can you scratch my back for me?" test). Take your right arm and reach your hand down your back as far as you can. At the same time, take your left arm and reach that hand up your back. Do your fingers meet? If they do, estimate how many inches they overlap.

Your Weight. A number of factors affect weight, including genes, which determine your body size and shape; the amount of exercise you get; your age and gender; and what and how much you eat. Your weight is a good number to note when you're beginning a plan to shape up, but it's not a magic number that automatically

HEART RATE

AGE	TARGET HR ZONE 50-75 % AVERAGE	MAXIMUM HEART RATE 100 %
55 years	83-123 beats per minute	165
60 years	80-120 beats per minute	160
65 years	78-116 beats per minute	155
70 years	75-113 beats per minute	150

Your maximum heart rate is approximately 220 minus your age.
The figures are averages and should be used as general guidelines.
Source: American Heart Association

pronounces whether or not you're in shape. Get on the scale; write down the total. (Don't worry, nobody's peeking.) Whether your weight is healthy depends primarily on your body composition, in other words how much of your weight is fat and how much is dense (like your bones and muscles and organs). The **Body Mass Index**, or BMI, measures your height and weight to help determine how much body fat you have. Power up your trusty calculator. It's math time. To calculate your BMI, divide your weight in kilograms by your height in meters squared.

Translated into U.S. measurements, your BMI is 705 times your weight in pounds, divided by your height in inches squared. Suppose you weigh 140 pounds and are 65 inches tall. Your BMI would be: 705 times 140, divided by 4,225 (65 inches squared), or 23.36, making you just fine.

Your Measurements. What's your waist-to-hip ratio? Where your fat is concentrated can signal danger. Whether you're a man or a woman, if you're apple-shaped, or fat around the middle, you risk more health problems than if you're pear-shaped, or heavy around the buttocks and thighs. To figure out your shape, stand up, exhale normally, then measure your waist at your belly button. Don't squeeze!! Note the measurement.

Next, measure your hips, circling the biggest part of your buttocks. Divide the waist measurement by the hip measurement and you get your waist-to-hip ratio. For example, if your waist measures 34 inches and your hips total 40 inches, divide 34 by 40 and you get a waist-to-hip ratio of 0.85.

WAIST-TO-HIP RATIO

	WOMEN	MEN
Favorable:	less than .80	less than .90
Borderline:	.80 to .85	.90 to 1.0
Unfavorable:	above .85	above 1.0

BMI

BMI OF...	MEANS YOU ARE...
18.5 or less	Underweight
18.5 – 24.9	Normal
25 – 29.9	Overweight
30 – 34.9	Obese

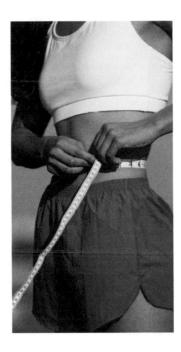

emotionally fit

Every body needs some buddy sometimes

For many people, coming to terms with their shape is the hardest part of improving it. Before you can start getting fit, you need to understand one more thing—why you're out of shape to begin with.

Get out that notebook again and make a list of everything you believe keeps you from shaping up. Do you feel you have to finish everything on your plate and everyone else's? Do you turn to food for solace? Do you eat the wrong stuff? Are your portions out of control? If you don't eat healthful foods, what's getting in the way? No time to shop or cook? You don't know what the heck you're supposed to eat to begin with? If you don't exercise, why don't you?

Once you list your obstacles, you can address them. First, accept the choices you have made in the past. Don't beat yourself up about them. Next, know and believe you can change your behavior. Now, start to change it. There are chapters in this book dedicated to losing weight, eating right, and exercising. Each will help you formulate a strategy for hurdling the obstacles you encounter.

How you tailor these plans is as unique as your fingerprint. You need to pinpoint what gets you motivated and what options match your personality, time constraints, and budget.

THE BUDDY SYSTEM

To help you in your fitness quest, hook up with a buddy. Your mate, your neighbor, a colleague, a friend, or a kindred spirit online can encourage you to get up, get moving, and eat right. You can exercise together, cook together, eat together, or plan your strategies together. You can turn to each other for help when things get rocky and help each other get back on track. If no buddy comes to mind, take a class; join a gym or a club; put a notice in the newsletter at work, the library, or your place of worship; or join a fitness community online.

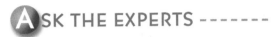

What causes most people to give up on a fitness program?
The number one reason people abandon their quest for good health is lack of time. But if you incorporate shaping up into your daily routine right from the start—making it as much a part of your day as brushing your teeth—you're less apt to drop out.

But I can never find spare time in the day.
Exactly. That's why you need to plan. Fitting in exercise and healthy eating is simply a matter of logistics. You build them into your schedule, like the kids' soccer practice and meetings with your boss. If you wait for "spare time" you may wait forever. Study your calendar and note where you have pockets of free time. Then pencil in appointments with yourself that will be dedicated to shaping up. These can be as diverse as going to the library to look for interesting exercise and healthy cooking videos, to climbing the Stairmaster for 40 minutes, to checking out the new gym in town.

EASE INTO IT

"I am healthy, trim, and strong." Write this affirmation on sticky notes and put them all over the place—on the fridge, in the car, on your computer monitor, and on the TV. Read it and believe it.

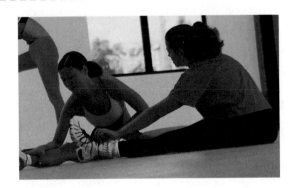

now what do I do?

Answers to common questions

Q I'm in pretty pathetic shape. Will I have to exercise to the point of exhaustion and starve myself every day to get in shape?

Not at all. As you'll learn later in this book, workouts don't have to be long and hard in order to reap the health benefits. Done on a regular basis, even a moderate amount of movement will improve your health tremendously. Eating what's good for you doesn't mean limiting your diet to fiber and grass. You can eat all kinds of fun, interesting, and delicious foods and still control your weight.

Q How can I ever get started?

You already have! By reading this far, you're on your way. Proceed slowly, and start making changes today—even if all you do is turn on your favorite radio station and dance around the room for one song; or you reach for the light popcorn instead of ice cream after dinner. Tomorrow, try to dance for two songs and eat a new vegetable. Add a couple of minutes to your exercise and healthy eating efforts each day.

Q There's no way I can find time to exercise. What do you suggest?

Finding time at first is challenging. To start, walk around your home or the parking lot at work for at least 5 to 10 minutes before work, again at lunchtime, and right after work. This gets you 15 to 30 minutes of movement during your day, in itty-bitty snippets of time that won't interfere with your day. It won't get you to ultimate cardiovascular fitness (which you'll learn about in *Exercising your options*), but it's a great start.

Q At first it's so hard to see results. How can I keep motivated?

Build in rewards. If you live for baseball games, watch them while you're exercising. No exercise, no ball game! Save the money you would otherwise spend on beer, nachos, ice cream, or donuts, and buy yourself a treat each week—a new CD, book, magazine, or massage. Make sure it's something you really enjoy. Most importantly, keep your eye on the prize—feeling, looking, and living great!

BOOKS

Strong Women Stay Slim, Miriam E. Nelson, Ph.D.
Primer on how weight, nutrition, fitness, and exercise work together. Includes logs and exercises.

Fat to Firm at Any Age, Alisa Bauman and Sari Harrar
Upbeat, positive strategies for eating, cooking, and exercising to attain a slim, healthy, and well-toned body.

Eating Well for Optimum Health, Andrew Weil, M.D.
A candid guide to what to eat, why to eat it, and how to prepare it. Dispels the myths of fad diets and offers a thorough primer on nutrition and health.

WEB SITES

www.shapeup.org
Tips from former Surgeon General C. Everett Koop on physical fitness and how to manage your weight safely.

www.cdc.gov/nccdphp/dnpd/index.htm
A government-sponsored Web site with lots of information on nutrition and fitness.

www.caloriecontrol.com
Useful tools include a calorie counter, BMI calculator, and an exercise calculator.

www.mayoclinic.com
Reliable in-depth news and information on diseases, illnesses, and nutrition. Recipe makeovers and a database of recipes.

PUBLICATIONS

The Wellness Letter
(800) 829-9080
www.berkeleywellness.com
Offers news and strategies on health and well-being. Put out by the University of California/Berkeley.

Prevention Magazine
(800) 813-8070
Articles on health, weight management, and fitness.

2

nutrition basics

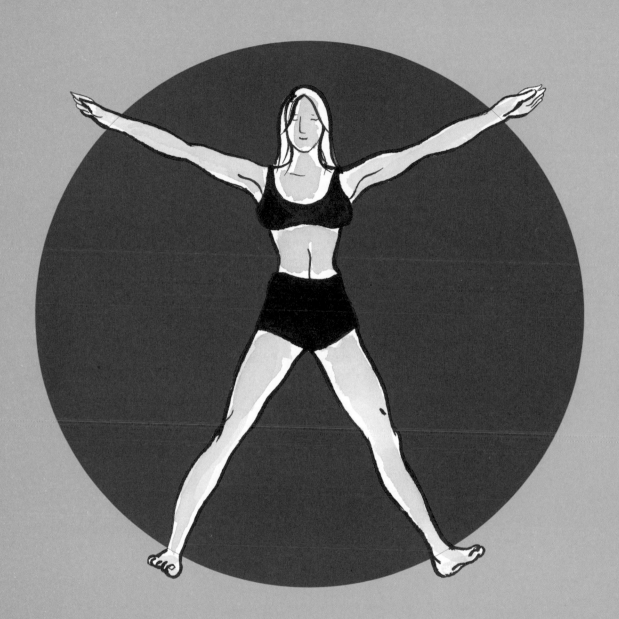

Managing and maintaining your weight
is an important aspect of living a long,
healthy life. Find out what your
healthy weight range should be and how
you can get there—safely.

nourishing your body

Learning the basics helps you make healthy choices

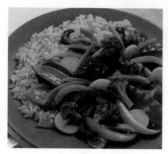

Eating is one of the joys of life. But to get the most out of life— to work productively, reduce your risk of disease, to look and feel great—you need to eat right. The path to eating right is simply knowing some basics about nutrition and making the right choices. To do that, you need a little knowledge.

Few of us ever learned how food really works in our bodies, or which foods and nutrients are best. Why do you need to know, you ask? After all, you don't need to know how a car works to drive it. But it's important to know what keeps your body working. That way, you'll finally understand why the experts keep saying, "A moderate, balanced, and varied diet will help keep you healthy and fit."

Good food and drink do more than just taste good. They provide your body with energy and nutrients that build, maintain, and repair tissues in every part of your body.

How does your body get what it needs from food? Depending on what you eat, your body breaks down food into various nutrients. Your body needs **macronutrients**, namely carbohydrates, fats, and proteins, to provide energy, and to build and maintain your tissues. It needs vitamins and minerals, called **micronutrients**, to vitalize all sorts of bodily functions. And your body needs water to keep every cell in you working properly.

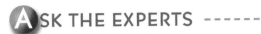

ASK THE EXPERTS

How do the nutrients in food actually work in my body?
Nutrients are absorbed from your intestines into your bloodstream and carried to the cells of your body, where they accomplish their amazing work.

I have no idea what I should eat to stay healthy. Do I need to take a nutrition course?
Not at all. Fortunately, there is plenty of guidance out there. For one, the Food and Nutrition Board of the Institute of Medicine has established Dietary Reference Intakes or DRIs. The DRIs recommend levels of nutrients that optimize health and maximum levels of some nutrients that can be consumed without toxic side effects. New DRIs are now replacing the RDAs, or Recommended Dietary Allowances, which spell out the levels of protein, vitamins, and minerals that are considered adequate to protect against deficiency.

Do I have to follow these recommendations to a T?
You don't have to adhere to them at every meal or even every day. Rather, use them to guide your food choices over the course of several days.

What's the food guide pyramid about?
The U.S. Department of Agriculture (USDA) has translated the RDAs and the DRI guidelines into recommendations for the kinds, and amounts, of food to eat each day. These appear in the Food Guide Pyramid. (More about the guidelines and the pyramid in *Chapter 4*.)

fueling up

You can count on calories for energy

Calories: You read them on food labels. You talk about them. You may count them—and even curse them.

What is a **calorie**? Technically speaking, a calorie is the amount of energy needed to raise the temperature of one gram of water by one degree centigrade. (Don't worry, you won't be tested on this!) In the real world, calories measure how much energy is in food and how much energy your body uses for growth, to maintain itself, and for physical activity. Take an apple, for example. The 81 calories in that apple produce 81 calories of energy.

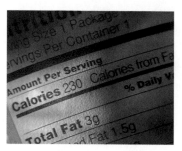

Digestion releases the carbohydrates, fat, and protein in the foods you eat. These nutrients are absorbed into your bloodstream and some are converted to **glucose** (blood sugar). The energy in glucose then enters your cells to fuel your body's work.

Carbohydrates, fats, and proteins contain different amounts of calories: 9 per gram of fat and 4 each per gram of carbohydrate and protein. A gram of alcohol provides 7 calories. Vitamins, minerals, water, cholesterol, and fiber have no calories.

Your body burns energy, even while it's at rest, for basic functions like breathing, regulating body temperature, and sending messages to your brain. The amount of energy your body spends on these functions is your **basal metabolic rate** (BMR), and it accounts for about 60 percent of the calories you need each day. An additional 30 percent of your calories fuels physical activity. The other 10 percent is used to digest and absorb nutrients.

To maintain your weight, the calories you take in must equal the number your body uses. Take in more calories than you expend, and you gain weight. Take in fewer calories than you expend, and you lose weight. Pretty simple, right?

How Many Calories Do You Need?

Your calorie needs depend on a few things:

Your age: The older you are, the fewer calories you need (about 2 percent less every 10 years after age 25). As you age, your body replaces muscle with fat, which burns fewer calories than muscle. The good news is that physical activity can help you keep more muscle mass.

Your gender: Men need more calories than women because they have 10 to 20 percent more muscle and less body fat than women.

Heredity and body size, shape, and composition: Your body is programmed to have a certain metabolic rate and body type. A lean, muscular body burns more calories than a soft, round body. A larger body requires more energy to move, so the more you weigh, the more calories you burn.

Your activity level: The longer, the harder, and the more frequently you work out, the more energy your body requires. Physical activity can actually boost your BMR for several hours after you exercise, helping you to burn even more calories.

The following formula gives you an estimate of how many calories you need each day to maintain your current weight.
- If you're sedentary, multiply your weight by 14
- If you're moderately active, multiply your weight by 17
- If you're active, multiply your weight by 20

Note: "Moderately active" means you participate in 3 to 4 aerobic sessions per week, and "active" means participating in 5 to 7 sessions.

sorting out the fats

Discover what happens when you chew the fat

A lot of what you hear about fat is negative. But fat is vital to your health. It is the most concentrated source of food energy, providing more than twice as many calories per gram as carbohydrates or protein. If not for fat, your body couldn't circulate, store, and absorb certain vitamins. Fat helps create cell walls, prevent skin dryness and flaking, and produces vitamin D and hormones such as estrogen. Body fat cushions and supports your internal organs, protects your nerve pathways, and provides insulation to keep you warm.

Fat makes foods more appealing by adding aroma, flavor, and texture (the creaminess of ice cream and the crispiness of French fries, for example). After a meal, fat helps you feel full because it stays in your stomach longer than carbohydrates and protein.

How could something that's so good be bad? Problems crop up when you eat too much and the wrong kinds of fat, which can lead to obesity, increased blood cholesterol levels, and heart disease.

Saturated fats and **trans fats** are the bad guys of the fat family. These fats can hike your blood cholesterol—even more than high-cholesterol foods do! Foods high in saturated fats include beef and whole milk dairy products, and processed foods made with coconut or palm oil. Cookies, crackers, snacks, and fast foods made with partially hydrogenated oils contain trans fats.

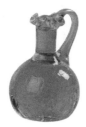

Unsaturated fats are either **monounsaturated** or **polyunsaturated**. These fats can help lower blood cholesterol levels when substituted for saturated fats. Foods high in monounsaturated fats include olive, peanut, and canola oil, as well as avocados and nuts. Corn, safflower, sunflower, cottonseed, and soybean oil are high in polyunsaturated fat.

Try to limit your fat intake to about 30 percent of your calories each day, and keep your saturated fats to less than 10 percent of your daily calories.

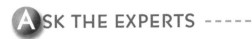

ASK THE EXPERTS

I thought cholesterol was bad, but my mother says I'm wrong. Who's right?

In this case, mother knows best. You need this waxy, fat-like substance that circulates in your bloodstream to help make hormones such as estrogen and testosterone, and to build and repair cells. Your body produces all the cholesterol you need, but certain foods and beverages give you additional cholesterol.

There are two main types of cholesterol in your blood: **low-density lipoproteins**, or LDLs, and **high-density lipoproteins**, or HDLs. LDL ("bad") cholesterol deposits fats and cholesterol on the walls of your arteries, forming a thick, fatty substance called plaque. Plaque can build up and narrow your arteries, restricting or even blocking blood flow. HDL ("good") cholesterol removes fat and cholesterol from your artery walls. High levels of HDL in your blood may prevent heart disease, while low HDL levels may promote heart disease.

How can I keep my blood cholesterol levels in check?

Try to limit your daily intake of dietary cholesterol to 300 milligrams. (Dietary cholesterol comes only from animal sources, such as the fat in dairy products, egg yolks, meats, poultry, and seafood.) But reducing the cholesterol in your diet is only part of the answer. Keep your fat intake within the recommended guidelines, paying particular attention to limiting saturated fat. Add fiber to your diet. And, get moving: Vigorous exercise can boost HDL and lower LDL levels. It also helps control weight, which also keeps cholesterol in check.

EASE INTO IT

To figure out the approximate amount of fat you should consume each day, multiply your daily calorie need (you calculated this earlier) by .30. Then, divide by 9 to convert to grams. For example, if you need 2,100 calories: 2,100 x .30 = 630 calories from fat. Now divide by 9 to convert to grams: 630 ÷ 9 = 70 grams. To find your saturated fat limit, multiply your daily caloric requirement by .10: 2,100 x .10 = 210 calories. Divide by 9 to convert to grams: 210 ÷ 9 = 23 grams of saturated fat.

building on protein

From growing hair to producing antibodies, protein is a pro

Every cell in your body packs protein. Enzymes, hormones, and antibodies are all proteins. When cells wear out, protein helps repair them, and when there is growth or healing, it helps make new tissue. Protein comes to the rescue as an emergency source of energy when carbohydrates and fat aren't available.

Protein consists of building blocks called amino acids. Like letters of the alphabet that combine to form words, amino acids combine to create tens of thousands of types of proteins, each with its own job. Your body makes some amino acids, called non-essential amino acids. Others, called essential amino acids, must come from your diet.

FITNESS FACTS

Soy: Oh, Boy!

Eating soy is an inexpensive and healthful way to get protein. If you substitute low-fat soy products for meat, you can lower the fat and cholesterol content of your diet. Soy contains phytochemicals (more about these later), which may reduce the risk of osteoporosis, a condition which gradually causes bones to become brittle, porous, and likely to fracture. Eating soy on a regular basis may lower your risk of developing cardiovascular disease and certain cancers. On top of that, soy consumption may decrease LDL cholesterol and fats in the blood and help prevent the hot flashes that can accompany menopause. Shoot for at least 25 grams of soy protein in your diet every day. One way to do this is to add soy products to the dishes you prepare. Soy foods include soybeans, tofu, soy milk, tempeh, and textured soy protein (an ingredient in many meat substitutes).

Some foods, like meat, fish, poultry, and dairy products have complete proteins, which means they supply adequate amounts of all the essential amino acids. Other protein sources, like grains, peas, beans, peanuts, nuts, seeds, and many vegetables, are incomplete because they lack one or more of the essential amino acids. But the amino acids in one incomplete protein can compensate for the missing amino acids in another. Take a peanut butter sandwich: The amino acids in the peanuts compensate for those missing in the bread, and vice versa. Vegetarians who eat no animal products can get all the essential amino acids by eating different plant foods throughout the day.

Most Americans consume more protein than they need. Consider this: A 3-ounce serving of lean meat (about the size of a deck of cards) supplies 21 grams of protein—about half of what many people need in a day! Eating too much protein can stress your kidneys as they try to eliminate the excess. When you choose protein foods, try to avoid sources high in saturated fats.

EASE INTO IT

A healthy adult needs .8 grams of protein each day per kilogram of body weight, or about .36 grams per pound. To figure out how much protein you need, take your weight and multiply it by .36. Say you weigh 130 pounds. You would need 47 grams of protein a day (130 x .36).

clarifying carbs

Unraveling the simple and complex story on carbohydrates

Carbohydrates, or carbs, are your body's main source of energy. Most carbohydrates come from plants, but dairy products also contain carbohydrates.

During digestion, carbs break down into three simple sugars. Glucose is the only simple sugar your body uses directly for energy; the others must be converted to glucose. Glucose immediately enters the bloodstream (that's why it's called blood sugar) to fuel your cells. Some glucose that isn't needed right away (in other words, when your blood sugar is high) is stored as a type of carbohydrate called **glycogen**; glucose that can't be stored is converted to fat. When your blood sugar is low, your body converts the glycogen to glucose.

There are two types of carbs, simple and complex. Most foods are a combination of both, but usually contain more of one type than the other.

Simple carbohydrates, which tend to taste sweet, occur either naturally (in fruits, milk products, honey, and some vegetables) or in processed form (table sugar, brown sugar, and corn syrup, for example). **Complex carbohydrates** are the starches in your diet. Complex carbs require more time and energy to digest than simple carbs, which means they make you feel full longer. Complex carbs

FITNESS FACTS

How Many Carbs?

A good bet is 45 to 65 percent of your daily calories should be carbohydrates. Take the caloric requirement you calculated and multiply it by .55 or .60. Then divide by 4 to convert to grams.

Sweet Stuff

Despite the bad rap that sugar gets, there's no evidence that it causes health problems other than tooth decay. Of the many sugars in your diet—refined white sugar, brown sugar, honey, fructose, corn syrup, or maple syrup, to name a few—none is any better or any worse than another. They all provide the same number of calories (15 calories in a teaspoon) but little nutritional benefit.

Keep in mind that foods with processed sugars may be high in fat and calories, and low in fiber, while foods with naturally occurring sugars supply vitamins, minerals, and sometimes fiber.

also help your body release insulin at a more constant and even rate, giving you more consistent energy and blood sugar levels. Whole grains, whole grain cereals, peas, beans, and potatoes all contain complex carbohydrates. Foods that are high in complex carbohydrates are also high in fiber (more about fiber in the next section).

It's best if the bulk of your carbs come from the complex variety in grains and from the natural sugars in fruits and vegetables.

fiber and water

Fiber and water do your body good

Dietary fiber packs plenty of benefits. **Soluble fiber** (it dissolves in water) may help lower LDL, or "bad," blood cholesterol in some people. Good sources of soluble fiber include oat bran, legumes, barley, citrus fruits, apples, and carrots.

FITNESS FACTS: WHETTING YOUR APPETITE

Here's one thing you can't live without. (No, not that last episode of *Survivor!*) It's water, probably the most important nutrient of all. Unfortunately, it's often taken for granted.

You can survive for weeks without food, but less than a week without water. Nearly every process in your body relies on water. It regulates your body temperature; carts off toxins and wastes; transports nutrients and oxygen to your cells; maintains blood volume (blood is about 80 percent water!); dissolves vitamins, minerals, and other nutrients; helps prevent constipation; and cushions your joints. Every part of your body—from cells to organs—requires water.

You lose about 10 cups of water every day—mostly through perspiration, urination, and bowel movements. Hot and humid temperatures, high altitudes, pregnancy and breastfeeding, working out, and eating a diet high in sodium, protein, or fiber boosts your need for water.

Drinking water is the best way to replenish the fluid you lose and avoid dehydration. Milk, juice, carbonated water, and decaffeinated tea and coffee also can fill your water requirement. Caffeinated and alcoholic beverages make you lose water. Fruits and vegetables contain water, but since it's difficult to measure how much, don't include them in your total.

Insoluble fiber (it doesn't dissolve in water) absorbs up to 15 times its weight in water, helping prevent constipation and some kinds of diarrhea. It adds bulk to and softens stools, which helps prevent diverticulosis and hemorrhoids. Find insoluble fiber in whole wheat and other whole grains, bran, cereals, vegetables (for example, cabbage, cauliflower, green beans, and potatoes), the skins of fruits and vegetables, root vegetables (carrots and beets), and foods with edible seeds, such as raspberries and strawberries.

Foods naturally rich in fiber boost your health in other ways. They contain vitamins and minerals, and are low in calories and fat. They often take longer to chew, which means you tend to eat less. What's more, their bulk makes you feel full longer, so you're less likely to overeat.

Aim for 21 to 38 grams of soluble and insoluble fiber daily, but not much more than that. Eating too much fiber moves food through your intestinal tract so quickly that nutrients—especially iron, zinc, and calcium—don't have time to get absorbed. If your diet is low in fiber now, up your fiber intake gradually to avoid diarrhea, gassiness, bloating, and abdominal pain. And be sure to drink more water as you eat more fiber.

EASE INTO IT

To figure out how much water you need, simply divide your weight in pounds by 2. If you weigh 160 pounds, for instance, you need 80 ounces, or 10 cups, of water daily. Hike your intake if it's hot, you work out, or if any of the factors on the previous page apply.

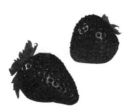

vitamins & minerals

Vitamins and minerals: small but mighty

Their names look like alphabet soup, but the truth is simple: Vitamins and minerals affect every process in your body. But they don't work alone. They team up with other nutrients to keep your body functioning normally.

Since your body can't produce most vitamins and minerals, you must get them from your diet. But be careful: Consuming too little of a vitamin or a mineral for prolonged periods puts you at risk of deficiency; consuming too much can be toxic.

Vitamins help trigger processes in your body, build tissue, and help derive energy from carbs, protein, and fat. To do their work, they often join forces with **enzymes**, proteins that make chemical reactions take place in your body.

There are two types of vitamins. **Water-soluble vitamins** dissolve in water, and are carried by your bloodstream throughout the body. Your body uses the vitamins it needs, then excretes most of the excess. (Even so, excessive amounts of these vitamins can harm you.) **Fat-soluble vitamins**—they dissolve in fat—travel through your bloodstream attached to chemicals made with fats (another reason you need fats in your diet). Instead of eliminating what you don't need, your body stores excess fat-soluble vitamins, which can build to toxic levels.

Minerals also help trigger body processes—from transporting oxygen and regulating your heartbeat to maintaining proper fluid and chemical balance—and supply components for enzymes and hormones. **Major minerals** are those you need in the greatest quantity; **trace minerals** are needed in smaller quantities.

The following chart lists the vitamins and minerals you need—based on the new Dietary Reference Intakes (DRI) discussed on page 27—their functions, recommended daily intakes, and, in some cases, age categories and amounts not to exceed. It also highlights good food sources.

VITAMINS

mg= milligrams
mcg= micrograms
IU= International Units

FAT-SOLUBLE VITAMINS

Vitamin A
Benefits: Helps grow and develop bones, skin, and teeth; helps maintain healthy vision, skin, and mucous membranes; is an antioxidant; may prevent or slow progress of macular degeneration
Food sources: Deep yellow and orange fruits; green, deep yellow and orange vegetables; fortified foods

Vitamin D
Benefits: Helps absorb and deposit calcium for healthy bones and teeth
Food sources: Fortified milk, fortified cereals

Vitamin E
Benefits: Helps form muscles, blood cells, lung and nerve tissue; is an antioxidant
Food sources: Poultry, seafood, vegetable oils, whole grains, wheat germ, green leafy vegetables, seeds, peanut butter, nuts, eggs, fortified cereals

Vitamin K

Benefits: Helps produce blood, bone, and kidney tissue, and also helps blood to clot

Food sources: Green leafy vegetables (e.g., spinach, broccoli), eggs, dairy products, oats, potatoes

WATER-SOLUBLE VITAMINS

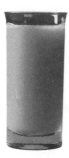

Vitamin C (ascorbic acid)

Benefits: Helps fight and resist infection, absorb iron, grow and maintain bones, teeth, ligaments, blood vessels, and gums, and heal wounds; is an antioxidant

Food sources: Citrus fruits and juices, peppers, broccoli, tomatoes, spinach, berries, melons, sweet potatoes, potatoes

Thiamin (vitamin B1)

Benefits: Helps convert carbohydrates into energy; helps nervous, muscular, and cardiovascular systems function

Food sources: Whole grains and cereals, enriched grain products, pork, legumes

Riboflavin (vitamin B2)

Benefits: Helps produce energy and maintain healthy skin, eyes, and nerve function

Food sources: Eggs, dairy products, poultry, meat, fish, whole or enriched grain products, dark-green leafy vegetables

Niacin (vitamin B3)

Benefits: Helps metabolize (use) carbs, protein, and fat; helps enzymes function

Food sources: Meat, poultry, seafood, fish, legumes, enriched or whole grains and cereals

Pantothenic Acid (vitamin B5)
Benefits: Helps metabolize carbs, fats, and protein, and manufacture adrenal hormones and chemicals for nerve function
Food sources: Meat, poultry, fish, whole grain cereals, legumes

Vitamin B6
Benefits: Helps produce proteins, red blood cells, hemoglobin, and insulin; helps metabolize and absorb protein; helps remove excess homocysteine (amino acid that may damage blood vessels and contribute to buildup of fatty plaque in arteries) from blood
Food sources: Poultry, fish, pork, nuts, whole grains, legumes, bananas, potatoes, spinach, prunes, watermelon

Vitamin B12
Benefits: Helps form red blood cells and amino acids, and maintain the central nervous system; builds genetic material
Food sources: Dairy products, eggs, meat, fish, poultry

Biotin
Benefits: Helps metabolize protein, fat, and carbohydrates, break down fatty acids, and synthesize genetic material
Food sources: Oats, poultry, meat, yeast, eggs, nuts, legumes, seeds, vegetables

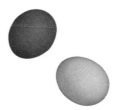

Folic Acid (folate)
Benefits: Helps synthesize genetic materials, form red blood cells and metabolize proteins; protects against heart disease and birth defects
Food sources: Dark green leafy vegetables, legumes, enriched grain products

MINERALS

MAJOR MINERALS

Calcium
Benefits: Helps build and maintain strong teeth and bones (helping to prevent osteoporosis), control blood pressure, contract muscles, conduct nerve impulses, and clot blood; may protect against stroke and lower risk of some cancers

Food sources: Dairy products, sardines (with bones), dark-green leafy vegetables, legumes, shellfish, fortified products, tofu

Fluoride
Benefits: Helps form bones and teeth and prevents tooth decay

Food sources: Seafood, tea, fluoridated water

Iron
Benefits: Helps transport oxygen in the bloodstream and transfer oxygen to muscles, protect against infection, and make proteins

Food sources: Red meat, fish, shellfish, nuts, dried fruit, dark-green vegetables, seeds, and fortified breads and cereals

Magnesium
Benefits: Helps build bones, teeth; helps muscular, nervous, and cardiovascular systems; is a component of many enzymes

Food sources: Legumes, nuts, whole grains, bananas, green leafy vegetables

Phosphorus

Benefits: Helps build strong bones and teeth, as well as genetic material, and helps to produce and store energy

Food sources: Meat, fish, eggs, dairy products, poultry, grain products, legumes

Potassium

Benefits: Helps maintain fluid balance, transmit nerve signals, and contract muscles

Food sources: Bananas, citrus fruits, dried fruits, potatoes, avocados, mushrooms, poultry, meat, fish, and milk

Sodium

Benefits: Helps maintain fluid balance and blood pressure, transmit nerve signals, and contract muscles

Food sources: Salt, processed foods, milk

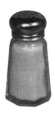

Zinc

Benefits: Promotes growth, tissue growth and repair; helps produce testosterone and metabolize nutrients

Food sources: Shellfish, meat, dairy products, wheat germ, whole grain products, legumes

TRACE MINERALS

Chromium

Benefits: Helps convert carbohydrates into energy

Food sources: Whole grain products, brewer's yeast, nuts, cheese

Copper

Benefits: Helps build bones, red blood cells, and hemoglobin

Food sources: Seafood, whole grain products, nuts, legumes

Iodine

Benefits: Is component of thyroid hormones
Food sources: Saltwater fish, milk, iodized salt, spinach

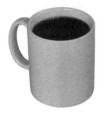

Manganese

Benefits: Helps metabolize carbohydrates and synthesize fats; aids bone development and brain function; is part of many enzymes
Food sources: Whole grain products, coffee, tea, green vegetables, fruits, nuts

Molybdenum

Benefits: Helps metabolize proteins; is component of many enzymes
Food sources: Dairy products, legumes, whole grain products, dark-green leafy vegetables

Selenium

Benefits: Is an antioxidant
Food sources: Seafood, poultry, meat, eggs, dairy products, whole grain products

Supplement Sense

Eating a well-balanced diet, with plenty of fruits, vegetables, and whole grains, will supply you with enough vitamins and minerals—not to mention other nutri- ents—so you don't need supplements. But if you're on a strict weight-loss diet, skip meals, eat foods high in sugar and 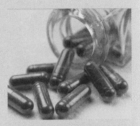 fat, suffer from digestive problems, take certain medications, or eat on the go, your diet may lack adequate amounts of vit- amins and minerals. Also, certain people—smokers (certainly not anyone reading this book!), pregnant and nursing women, the elderly, and vegetarians—may need additional vitamins and minerals. In these cases, it may make sense to take a sup- plement. Consult your physician or a registered dietitian first. Unless directed by your physician, don't exceed 100 percent of the Daily Values listed on the supplement labels. Check the expiration date on the bottle and beware of claims not backed by scientific evidence.

boosting immunity

The radical benefits of phytochem- icals and antioxidants

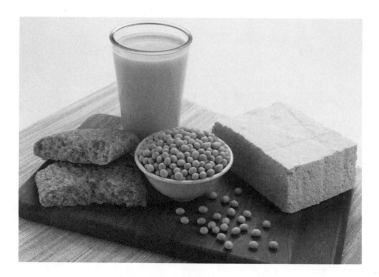

Leaf through an article on nutrition and you're bound to find something about substances in plants called **phytochemicals**. They protect plants from environmental threats—and may protect you from heart disease, some cancers, and other chronic health problems.

Some phytochemicals may block cancer-causing damage to your cells and lower blood cholesterol. Find them in **cruciferous vegetables** (broccoli, cauliflower, kale, Brussels sprouts, cabbage, bok choy, collard and turnip greens), garlic, and onions. Others, called **phytoestrogens**, may give women the benefits of estrogen, promoting cardiovascular health and healthy bones as well as relieving hot flashes. Look for these in soybeans, soy milk, tofu, tempeh, soy flour, and flaxseed, as well as in whole grains, beans, peas, and greens.

Some phytochemicals are antioxidants, which may protect against cancer, cardiovascular disease, infertility, cataracts, and problems associated with aging, and may also help lower blood pressure and blood cholesterol levels. What's their secret? They may neutralize some of the damage caused by free radicals, toxic substances produced when your body's cells burn oxygen for energy (and from environmental factors like pollution).

Vitamins C and E as well as substances called **carotenoids** are the best-known free-radical fighters. Carotenoids are the pigments that give fruits and vegetables their red, orange, and deep-yellow colors. There are three main types: **beta-carotene, lycopene,** and **lutein.** Foods rich in beta-carotene include winter squash, sweet potatoes, cantaloupe, pumpkins, mangoes, apricots, and carrots. Tomato products such as tomato sauce and paste, tomato soup, and ketchup are excellent sources of lycopene. (The lycopene in fresh tomatoes is not absorbed well; cook them in a little oil to aid absorption.) Good sources of lutein are broccoli, Brussels sprouts, spinach, kale, and egg yolk. If you're a tea drinker, take heart: Antioxidants in black and green tea may protect against cardiovascular diseases and cancer.

reading labels

Use labels to make wise food choices

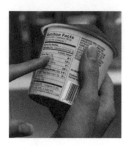

Reading food labels won't give you the thrills and chills of a spy novel, but it will help you make wholesome food choices. The labels, mandated by the Food and Drug Administration in 1994, take the guesswork out of shopping and eating. They tell you what's in a food product, and give you the tools to compare how one product stacks up against another.

When you read food labels, focus on the big picture. Don't worry if you get half the fat you should consume in a day from a couple of servings. It's the quality of your diet over several days, not one meal or one day, that matters.

Take a look at the sample label from a box of pasta on the next page.

   1. Serving Size: Similar products have similar serving sizes, so you can compare the nutritional value of different brands. Your actual serving may be larger.

2. Calories: Total calories in one serving.

3. Calories from Fat: Calories of fat in one serving.

4. Percent Daily Value: The percentage of nutrients, fat, and fiber, as well as the amount of sugar and protein, that one serving contributes to a 2,000-calorie diet (similar to the RDAs). Your calorie needs may be more or less than 2,000. The Daily Values are based on a diet with 30 percent of calories from fat (10 percent from saturated fat), 60 percent from carbohydrates, 10 percent from protein, with 12.5 grams of dietary fiber per 1,000 calories. For total fat, saturated fat, cholesterol, and sodium (especially if you have high blood pressure), the lower the percentage, the better. For fiber, the higher the percentage, the better.

5. Percent Daily Value: The most important vitamins and minerals. Shows the maximum recommended amounts of fat, saturated fat, cholesterol, and sodium, as well as the recommended amounts of carbohydrates and fiber in daily diets of 2,000 and 2,500 calories. Note that Daily Values for cholesterol and sodium stay the same, regardless of your calorie level.

Nutrition Facts

1 Serving Size 2 oz dry or 1 cup cooked
Servings Per Container 8

Amount Per Serving

2 Calories 200

3 Calories from Fat 10

	% Daily Value*
4	
Total Fat 1g	2%
Saturated Fat 0g	0%
Cholesterol 0mg	0%
Sodium 0mg	0%
Total Carbohydrate 40g	13%
Dietary Fiber 2g	8%
Sugars 1g	
Protein 7g	

5 Vitamin A	0%	Vitamin C	0%
Calcium	0%	Iron	10%
Thiamin	35%	Riboflavin	15%
Niacin	15%	Folate	30%

*Percent Daily Values are based on a 2,000-calorie diet. Your daily values may be higher or lower depending on your calorie needs.

		2,000	2,500
Calories		2,000	2,500
Total Fat	Less than	65g	80g
Saturated Fat	Less than	20g	25g
Cholesterol	Less than	300mg	300mg
Sodium	Less than	2,400mg	2,400mg
Total Carbohydrate		300mg	375mg
Dietary Fiber		25g	30g

Calories per gram:
Fat 9   Carbohydrate 4   Protein 4

Ingredients: Semolina, niacin, iron (ferrous sulfate), thiamine mononitrate, riboflavin, folic acid.

keeping a food diary

Discover what you eat— and why

Congratulations! You've learned what your body needs—and doesn't need. Now it's time to explore your diet. The best way to do this is to keep a food diary. Discover precisely what you're eating. Discover how much you eat. Discover why you eat. You might ask, is this a new form of torture? Not at all. If you're like most people, this can be a real eye-opener! Your food diary helps you determine if your diet is balanced, varied, and moderate. It's a tool to pinpoint trouble spots.

Take out that notebook you started in Chapter 1. Choose three days that represent your typical eating patterns: two weekdays and a weekend day. Each time you eat or drink anything, jot down exactly what it is, the time, the circumstances (snack during TV show, lunch with clients, for example), how hungry you were (use a scale of 0-5, with 5 being ravenous), and—don't forget this one—the reason you ate or drank (boredom, loneliness, socializing, anxiety, mealtime, hunger and so on). See the sample on the next page.

After three days:
Count up the calories, protein, fat, carbohydrate, fiber, vitamins, and minerals you ate and drank during the three days. You can use the information on food labels to assess the nutrients in the food or use an online calorie counter (see www.caloriecontrol.com or www.nal.usda.gov/fnic/foodcomp/). Now divide the total of the three days by 3 to get your daily average. Then see how that compares with the recommendations. Don't get discouraged if you discover your diet isn't what it could be. The next two chapters show you how to manage your weight and eat more healthfully.

WEDNESDAY

7:30 a.m. Stopped at the bakery for a low-fat blueberry muffin.

8:05 a.m. Coffee (with about a tbsp. of cream). Feeling famished—hunger level is 5. Spilled coffee on my suit while I was driving. Another trip to the cleaners . . .

10:15 a.m. On the way back from Rob's office, grabbed another cup of coffee (cream again).

1:45 p.m. Meeting with my client ran through lunch. She liked my presentation. Now I have to deliver. No time for lunch. Stopped at the vending machines and scarfed down a 2-ounce bag of Cheese Crunchies and a can of diet cola. Hunger level: 5. Cheese is nutritious, isn't it? Ate an apple at my desk.

3:20 p.m. It was Charlene's birthday, so Alex brought in a carrot cake—with cream cheese frosting. It was so good, I had two slices. Feeling hungry (4) and stressed. Washed down the cake with a cup of water from the cooler.

5:45 p.m. Got home from work. Feeling sort of hungry (3), so I ate a banana while I went through the mail—and enjoyed the peace and quiet.

6:30 p.m. Thank goodness—Hank picked up a box of fried chicken and mashed potatoes after he picked up the kids. Put a bowl of raw baby carrots out. Hunger: about a 3. I had a chicken breast (ate the yummiest part, the skin), potatoes with gravy (about half a cup), and seven baby carrots. Drank a glass and a half of water. Finished the potatoes on the kids' plates.

now what do I do?

Answers to common questions

Q What's the difference between an "enriched" food and a "fortified" food?

Both terms mean that nutrients were added to the food to make it more healthful. In enriched foods, nutrients lost during processing are added back. Fortified foods contain nutrients that weren't originally in the product. Sometimes, the terms "enriched" and "fortified" are used interchangeably on food labels.

Q My wife tells me I shouldn't use so much salt. What's the story?

Your wife may have a point. Many Americans consume more than 6 teaspoons of salt each day! (Most of the salt Americans consume doesn't come from salt shakers, but from processed and prepared foods.) For some people, a high-sodium (sodium is a component of salt) diet may increase the risk of high blood pressure, stroke, and kidney disease. Eating a diet low in sodium has been shown to improve high blood pressure. Check food labels. If you see the words salt, soda, or sodium, the product contains sodium. Try to limit your daily sodium consumption to 2,400 milligrams—a little more than one teaspoon of salt.

Q Should I be concerned about getting enough calcium?

Maybe. American adults, on average, get only about half the calcium they need. Calcium deficiency can lead to osteoporosis, muscle cramps, sleeplessness, and heart palpitations; it also has been linked to an increased risk of colon cancer and high blood pressure. During times of growth and as you get older, calcium is especially important. After the age of 65 or so, your calcium absorption decreases and you make less vitamin D, which helps absorb calcium. And as women age, their level of estrogen, which slows the loss of calcium in their bones, drops.

The best way to obtain calcium is from your diet. But if you don't get enough (if, for example, you cannot tolerate milk products), consider a supplement. Don't take more than 500 mg at a time, as your body absorbs small doses better. And be sure to get enough vitamin D. Do this is by exposing your skin to sunlight 10 to 30 minutes a day, or consider a multivitamin with vitamin D.

BOOKS

The American Dietetic Association's Complete Food and Nutrition Guide, Roberta Larson Duyff

Information on nutrients; healthy eating; maintaining a healthy weight; food safety; healthy cooking and eating out; nutrition for children, pregnant women, athletes, vegetarians, and older adults; food sensitivities; and eating disorders.

The Complete Book of Food Counts, Corrine T. Netzer

The nutritional content of more than 12,000 foods—generic, brand-name, fresh, frozen, and fast-food items—including calories, protein, carbohydrates, fat, fiber, cholesterol, and sodium.

Dr. Art Ulene's Complete Guide to Vitamins, Minerals, and Herbs, Art Ulene, M.D.

What vitamins, minerals, and herbs can do to prevent disease and improve health; how to obtain them; toxicity and deficiency; and designing a personalized supplement program.

Nutrition for Dummies, Carol Ann Rinzler

A guide to nutrition; healthy eating and cooking; food safety; food allergies; food processing and additives; fad diets, eating disorders, and eating out.

WEB SITES

www.caloriecontrol.com

Personal tools to calculate the number of calories per serving and keep track of total daily calorie consumption; how many calories you burn with dozens of activities; and Body Mass Index.

www.cyberdiet.com

Tools to calculate calories, grams of protein, carbohydrate, and fat (various types), as well as amounts of fiber, cholesterol, vitamins, and minerals; calories burned by activity; nutrient content of foods, including fast food; and nutrition news and facts.

www.navigator.tufts.edu

A rating and review guide of nutrition information on the Internet, developed by the Tufts University School of Nutrition Science and Policy.

www.webmd.com

Practical information and live events on weight control.

eating right

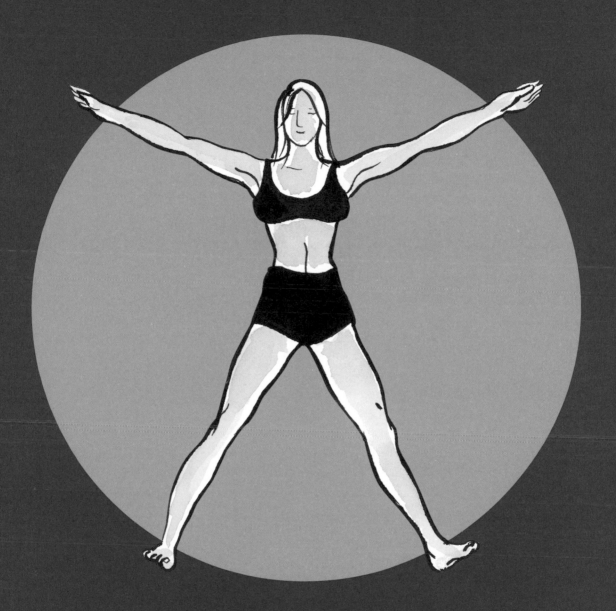

Unlock the secrets of the food pyramid.
The concept is simple, once
you begin making the right choices at the
supermarket, mealtime will be a snap.

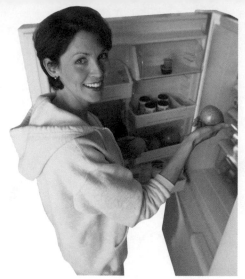

the right stuff

You'll salivate over these reasons to eat right

Eating right isn't something you have to force yourself to endure. It's a pleasure that offers a lifetime of benefits. It's like plugging your body directly into an energy source. The right foods power your brain to fuel decisions at work, generate energy to share with loved ones, and contribute to a nimble and strong body that is able to take you through life's paces.

By eating right you help shrink cholesterol, sugar, and blood pressure levels. You help reduce the risk of heart disease, headaches, digestive ailments, gallbladder disease, and many forms of cancer.

When your body has the food and nutrients it needs, you're less likely to get haunted by cravings. Better still, you're more alert and less irritable.

When you walk the path to healthful eating, you don't feel guilty about what you eat. Instead, you feel healthy, satisfied, and nourished—benefits that last a lifetime.

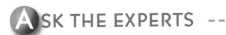

ASK THE EXPERTS

What's the secret formula to getting all these benefits, and how much is it going to cost?

There are no magical meals that you must ingest, no mysterious formulas to calculate, nothing to weigh, no potion to buy. You tailor what to eat according to your favorite foods, available time, budget, and interest (or lack thereof) in the kitchen. Eating well is practical and easy to figure out. There are some great tips in the following pages.

How about if I just eat a lot less? Won't that help me shape up?

Ironically, when consumption falls too low, your body thinks it's starving and clicks into conservation mode. This screeches your metabolism to a crawl in order to preserve the sparse calories you've fed it. You don't want this to happen! So, instead, keep your body running all day long by eating small, healthful snacks in addition to your three squares a day.

If I exercise, won't I get all these benefits without having to scrutinize everything I eat?

While exercise certainly helps clear the path to getting in shape, it can't work miracles by itself. For example, you'd have to walk for two hours to cancel out the calories in one piece of pecan pie. Besides, exercise doesn't supply any nutrients your body needs. If you want to shape up, you must eat healthfully *and* exercise.

what to eat

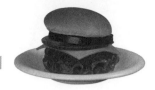

Simple guidelines for success

Your girlfriend goads you to drink more milk. Your dad packs in the protein and your sister starts the day with a soy shake. Your brother won't eat anything that's not organic. Your mother measures every mouthful and your cousin counts her carbohydrates. With all the fads out there, it's no wonder you can't figure out what to eat!

You don't need to tether yourself to a food scale, swear yourself to soy, or understand chemistry to unlock the secrets of healthful eating. You don't have to eat boring green things, or bread that tastes like cardboard, either. In fact, you can butter your bread, bake cookies with the kids, eat a cheeseburger at the company picnic, and still stay on track.

FITNESS FACTS

Digesting the Latest Headlines

Just when you think you have it figured out, along comes another study, diet book, or food guru telling you you've got it all wrong. How can you judge a new report for yourself? First, check to see who's behind the information. (University and government studies tend to be objective. Surveys by special interest groups may reflect a special agenda.) Read the entire story, not just the attention-grabbing headline. Determine how the study compares to previous findings. (Legitimate reports will always compare the survey's findings to previous beliefs.) Does the article include comments and responses from credible sources such as the USDA, the American Dietetic Association, or university spokespeople?

Note the number of people studied and their physical makeup. Are they like you in terms of gender, age, and weight? If there are no numbers or statistics cited, the survey could have included a handful of people whose physical makeup is a far cry from yours, or laboratory animals.

Don't change eating habits on the basis of one study if that's all you have to support the findings. Call your local hospital or university, ask for the nutrition department, and find out what they have to say about the report. Many will be happy to discuss the findings with you.

Food That Makes You Fat

Contrary to popular belief, no one food automatically makes you fat! Your body stores excess carbohydrates, fat, or protein as fat no matter whether it comes from a bagel or the cream cheese on top of it. If you eat a lot of fat, you'll likely put on the pounds faster though, as a gram of fat packs more than twice as many calories as a gram of carbohydrates or protein. To avoid plumping up, keep your caloric intake consistent with the calories you expend.

The USDA's *Dietary Guidelines for Americans* spells out the recipe for healthful eating. The blueprint calls for you to aim for a healthy weight and to be physically active each day. Also:

- Eat a variety of foods to provide the more than 40 nutrients your body needs. Choose whole grains, fruits, and vegetables each day, as no one food provides all the nutrients you need.

- Make sensible, healthful choices. Choose a diet low in saturated fat and cholesterol. About 30 percent of calories should come from total fat, and no more than 10 percent from saturated fat.

- Choose a diet moderate in sugars, salt, and sodium. If you drink alcoholic beverages, do so in moderation.

- Keep food safe to eat.

the food pyramid

Do your selections stack up?

You don't need to scour the Internet, pore over cooking magazines, or examine diet books to uncover the secret to healthful eating. Chances are the formula is hidden in your cupboards somewhere. Check out the back of a cereal box or a carton of milk. You may see a picture or drawing of a pyramid of different foods. If you haven't looked at it in a while, take time to review it because the **Food Guide Pyramid** shows you what to eat.

The USDA constructed the pyramid to help identify the building blocks of healthful eating without having to count grams or follow some guru. A quick look confirms that no food is off limits. Instead, the pyramid suggests how many servings to eat on a given day from the five food groups: grains, fruits, vegetables, milk/dairy products, and meat/proteins. Foods within each group contain similar nutrients and contribute to the body in a unique way.

While the pyramid illustrates what types of foods to consume, it doesn't tell you which are better than others. Not all foods within a group are created equally, so scaling the pyramid can be a bit precarious. In fact, the pyramid is currently being revised to provide better guidance.

To make the smartest selections, stick with foods that pack the most nutrients and are lower in fat. For example, a piece of white bread or a hot dog bun could conceivably count as a serving in the grain group. However, these selections pale in comparison to whole grains, which are loaded with nutrients and fiber. Pass up the white stuff and go for a whole grain roll.

HERE'S HOW THE PYRAMID STACKS UP: EVERY DAY EAT...

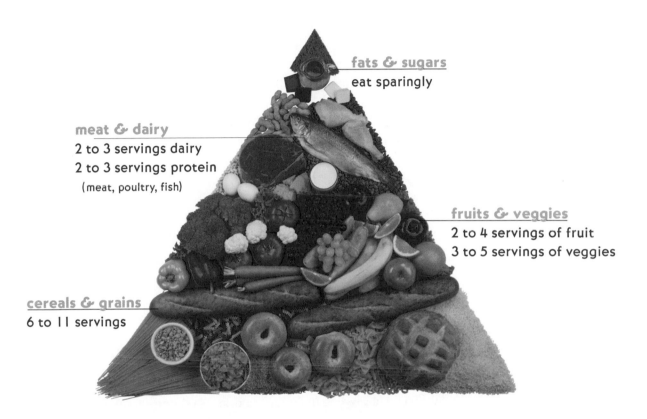

fats & sugars
eat sparingly

meat & dairy
2 to 3 servings dairy
2 to 3 servings protein
(meat, poultry, fish)

fruits & veggies
2 to 4 servings of fruit
3 to 5 servings of veggies

cereals & grains
6 to 11 servings

FITNESS FACTS

Eating by the Numbers

While the pyramid doesn't spell out the percentage of carbohydrates, protein, and fat you should aim for, you learned in *Nutrition Basics* that 45 to 65 percent of your total calories should come from complex carbohydrates. About 30 percent should come from fat, and less than 10 percent should come from saturated fat.

...grains, fruits, vegetables

Grains form the base of the pyramid's foundation. These include bread, cereal, rice, and pasta. This group supplies carbohydrates, B vitamins, minerals and, when you make the right selections, high fiber. You're supposed to eat 6 to 11 servings of grains each day. While this may seem like a lot, the key is in the serving size. For example, half a cup of cooked pasta is one serving, as is half an English muffin, one pancake, a slice of bread, or one ounce of dry cereal.

Grains Tip: Choose whole grain breads, cereals, and pastas over white or refined versions. Swap brown rice for white. Sprinkle whole grain cereal in your pancake mix, cottage cheese, or yogurt. Try a new grain, such as barley or quinoa.

Fruits and vegetables form separate building blocks in the pyramid. On the fruit side, aim for two to four servings. For the veggies, eat at least three to five servings. Fruits and veggies fill you up, nourish you with vitamins (especially A and C), taste great, are easy to prepare, fight cancer and heart disease, and help prevent osteoporosis. They're low in fat and calories. And, they crank up fiber intake. When you fill up with fruits and vegetables, there's less room for fatty foods.

Vary your choices of fruits and vegetables to ensure proper nutrition. If you eat an orange every day, you get the vitamin C you need, but may do so at the expense of another nutrient. Add in a mango and boost your vitamin A. Toss in a banana and power up your potassium. (Combine the three and you get a tasty fruit salad!)

Vegetables take a bit more planning. Chop some peppers and fold them into scrambled eggs; munch on carrot sticks on the way back from the gym; dip some broccoli, pea pods, or carrots into fat-free plain yogurt while you're cooking dinner; top your baked potato with salsa; or have some vegetable soup for lunch.

But what's a serving here? For vegetables, it's one cup raw, a half cup cooked, or 3/4 cup of juice. It's one medium potato, a cup of bean soup, two broccoli spears, half a cup of tomato sauce, or eight baby carrots. For fruits, it's one medium-size fruit (such as an apple or pear), half a large mango, 12 grapes, 1/2 cup of berries, a 3-inch melon wedge, 3/4 cup of fruit juice, or 1/4 cup of dried fruit.

Food for Thought

What you might consider a serving can be a whole lot larger than the one recommended by the pyramid. Consider that one serving of pasta is 1 ounce dry or 1/2 cup cooked. That means a one-pound box contains eight cups cooked, or 16 servings. So if a family of four sits down and splits a one-pound box of pasta, each person eats four servings! If you're trying to estimate servings of spaghetti on your plate at Aunt Josephine's Sunday dinner, but Auntie considers the mere notion sacrilegious, don't quiz her about ounces and servings. Use your fist as a guide. The average clenched fist equals about a cup, which is two servings.

Serving size can be the culprit when you change your diet but don't lose weight. For example, you sit down to a dinner of skinless baked chicken, pasta, steamed vegetables, a whole wheat roll, and fruit salad. You figure you're on the road to getting in shape. But the chicken's so tasty you eat a bit more, say a total of 6 oz. That's a **double** serving. Your two cups of pasta count as four servings of grains. (The roll counts as another.) The fruit salad is delightful—heck, it's fruit, you figure, how bad can another bowlful be? Those two bowls may exceed your recommended fruit servings for the day!

...dairy, meats, nuts

The milk, yogurt, and cheese group sits high up in the pyramid along with the meat, poultry, fish, dry beans, eggs, and nuts group. Therefore, you only need a couple of servings (two to three of each group, at the most) to get the daily nutrition you need.

Dairy products provide calcium, protein, vitamins, and minerals. What's a serving of this group? A cup of milk or yogurt, 1 1/2 ounces of unprocessed cheese, 2 ounces of processed cheese, or 3/4 cup of cottage cheese all equal one serving. (No way to measure those chunks of cheese at a party? Use your thumb. From the tip to the knuckle is about one ounce.)

Beware of your selections! When choosing whole milk dairy products, you clog up your system with extra calories, cholesterol, and saturated fat. Go with low-fat or no-fat versions and you enjoy the same terrific source of calcium, protein, and vitamins D and B12, without the gunk.

Dairy Tip: Choose low- and no-fat versions of cottage cheese, yogurt, and milk. Note that calcium is found in many vegetables, including kale, collards, and broccoli, in tofu, and in some fortified orange juices, cereals, and breads.

In the pyramid group featuring meats through nuts, you find great sources of protein, lots of B vitamins, and minerals like iron and zinc. One serving of cooked lean meat, fish, or skinless poultry is two to three ounces (about the size of the palm of your hand). A can of tuna? Though a 6-ounce can fits in your hand, it counts as 2 1/2 servings. A half cup of cooked legumes, one egg, or two tablespoons of peanut butter each count as a third of a serving.

The meat group is a prime example of why you need to scrutinize your selections. A 6-ounce hamburger uses up nearly your entire daily serving allocation and is full of fat and cholesterol. An egg counts as one ounce of lean meat, but it's full of cholesterol. When choosing meats, select lean cuts (look for those tabbed loin or round), and remove the skin from chicken or turkey before you eat it. (If you skin it before you cook it, the meat will dry out. Don't worry, the meat won't absorb the fat.) Beef up your fish consumption, especially fish high in omega-3 fatty acids. Enjoy nuts; they are packed with fiber and nutrients.

Protein Tip: Eat more legumes, like lentils, peas, beans, and soybeans. They have no saturated fat or cholesterol; they're packed with protein, nutrients, and fiber, and are simple to prepare.

...fats, oils, sweets

It's dangerous high atop the pyramid, where fats, oils, and sweets lurk, as these can blindside you right off the path to healthy eating. It's not that you must stamp out fats—they help fuel muscles and transport some types of vitamins—but you get more bang for your caloric buck when deriving energy from protein and carbohydrates.

There is no serving requirement for fats. The pyramid simply instructs you to use them sparingly. Fats should account for about 30 percent of the day's total calories. Saturated fats (see page 30) shouldn't account for more than 10 percent or one-third of that 30 percent fat allowance.

Fat Tip: Many foods contain fats and sugars in their natural state, even when you don't add to them. These substances lie in ambush in butter, salad dressing, oil, margarine, soft drinks, mayonnaise, candies, corn syrup, cakes, honey, cream sauces, and some muffins.

Drink Up!

The Food Guide Pyramid leaves out a major component of solid nutrition—liquid. *Nutrition Basics* filled you in on the benefits of drinking water. Not drinking enough water leads to fatigue, dry skin, constipation, and often, the nagging feeling that you're hungry, when you're actually thirsty. Drinking water fills you up, too. It's a very important aspect of any plan to shape up.

Each day your body uses about 10 cups of water (more if you exercise, are in hot or cold temperatures, on an airplane, or are pregnant or nursing). You need to drink at least eight cups to replace them. (Water from food makes up the balance.) Note that juices and milk include water, so these beverages can count toward the total.

However, alcohol, tea, and coffee don't count! In fact, they stimulate your kidneys to produce urine, which actually dehydrates the body. Try not to drink too much of these beverages. Alcohol jacks up calorie intake and increases the risk of high blood pressure, heart disease, stroke, birth defects, and accidents. One 12-ounce bottle of beer equals 150 calories. (The higher the proof, the more calories.) Alcohol also reduces your resolve. Remember, always drink in moderation.

If you absolutely must have a cup of coffee or tea in the morning to jump-start the day, make sure to switch to decaf after the first cup.

Beware of coffeehouse drinks like mochaccino, hot chocolate, cappuccino, and the like. Depending on the contents, a mochaccino can pack more fat than a brownie à la mode. To slim down your selection, ask for skim milk and hold the whipped cream.

Kick the diet soda habit. Many contain unnatural additives and sodium—which make you feel thirsty and bloated. Regular soda is loaded with sugar—empty calories that don't contribute toward your health. If you're a soda fiend, wean yourself from this unhealthful choice by drinking sparkling water with a splash of fruit juice.

designing your food plan

Creating a program that appeals to your tastes

Sometimes it helps to know ahead of time exactly what you will put in your mouth and when. That's one reason some diets are so popular—they spell out exactly what you can eat and when. But you can't live the rest of your life toting around a diet book to figure out what and when you should eat something. To have long-term success, you need a new way of eating—not a diet. You need meals unique to your needs, with foods you enjoy, that are convenient for you to prepare within your time and budget.

Why not make a realistic plan? Sketch out a menu for a week. Try to plan three meals a day and at least one snack. Note the times you plan to eat. Make sure the servings fit the pyramid, and assess the nutritional content (you learned how in *Nutrition Basics*). Meals should match your time limitations. If you don't have an hour to chop, slice, cook, eat, and clean up, don't plan a dish that requires that much effort.

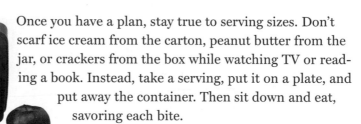

Once you have a plan, stay true to serving sizes. Don't scarf ice cream from the carton, peanut butter from the jar, or crackers from the box while watching TV or reading a book. Instead, take a serving, put it on a plate, and put away the container. Then sit down and eat, savoring each bite.

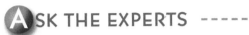

ASK THE EXPERTS

**I can't imagine not including my favorite foods in my plan.
What should I do?**

By all means, include foods that give you pleasure. Just keep portions in check. If you go overboard on something, make adjustments elsewhere in the day. If you love pasta, for example, and want to have a generous portion of it for dinner, cut back on grains at your other meals. If you're looking forward to celebrating your anniversary with filet mignon and chocolate soufflé at a favorite French restaurant, lighten up on the rest of the week's fare and enjoy the celebration. Just be sure to eat a variety of foods, so you won't limit your nutrients or overdo one nutrient at the expense of another.

**I have so many decisions to make in a day that figuring out what
to cook for dinner is one I can do without. Any suggestions?**

Sure! Ask a registered dietitian, a nutritionist, or a personal chef for help. Each will design meals for you and your family. The chef will even cook them for you at a cost that's often less than what you'd spend for take-out food. To find a registered dietitian in your area, call the American Dietetic Association's Consumer Nutrition Hot Line at (800) 366-1655 and ask for a referral, visit their Web site at **www.eatright.org**, or call your local social service agency.

pumping up your plan

Nutrition à la carte

Now is the time to really sink your teeth into what you eat. Give yourself the opportunity to make changes that set the stage for a lifetime of healthful eating. When planning menus:

Be creative. If you drag the same old turkey-on-whole-wheat to work each day, you're apt to run to the vending machine salivating over the Cheez Snax. (And you'll limit nutrients.) Expand your repertoire, visually and nutritionally.

Hike fiber intake. Include pears, raspberries, barley, whole wheat bread, and a host of high-fiber multigrain breakfast cereals. Try to eat at least four servings a week of legumes such as beans, peas, and lentils. A big bowl of bean, pea, or lentil soup takes care of a couple of servings. Add cooked beans or lentils to your pasta or rice dishes, or put them in the food processor and spread on whole wheat crackers or pita bread. Try bean or lentil salad, vegetable chili, and low-fat versions of refried beans, baked beans, and bean burritos.

Each day, aim for at least one fruit or vegetable that contains beta carotene (examples include carrots, sweet potatoes, squash, tomatoes, cantaloupes, and apricots), and another that's rich in vitamin C (like oranges, grapefruit, papayas, red peppers, broccoli, and tomatoes).

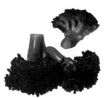 **Pencil in something from the cabbage family** at least a couple of times a week. Broccoli, collard and turnip greens, arugula, watercress, and other cruciferous vegetables help protect against certain types of cancer.

menu

Breakfast

Don't skip it. A solid breakfast is the best way to fuel up for the day. Include a little protein to keep you satiated following the meal.

Bypass the whole milk in favor of low-fat or skim. Use low- or no-fat yogurt or buttermilk when making pancakes or waffles. (In spite of its name, buttermilk is low in fat.)

In omelets or scrambled eggs, eliminate an egg yolk and add diced vegetables.

Put diced fruit on whole grain cereal or add it to a pancake or muffin mix.

Lunch

Eliminate the mayo and incorporate vegetables. Turkey on whole grain toast sounds **bo-o-o-ring**, but stick half a red pepper and a tablespoon of plain, no-, or low-fat yogurt into the food processor and you end up with a tasty and healthy sandwich spread. Add a couple of pea pods in the sandwich for added nutrients and some crunch.

Sneak in legumes. Mash up leftover beans (or open a new can) and spread a thin layer on toasted pita bread sprinkled with feta cheese and something green and crunchy, like lettuce, arugula, or thin pepper strips.

Rediscover soup. It's filling and full of things you might not eat otherwise, like navy beans or kale. Stay away from cream-based and cheese-filled soups, though, as they're loaded with fat.

Dinner

Eat fish a couple of times a week, especially cold-water fish like salmon and albacore tuna because they contain the good omega-3 fats.

Go vegetarian for a night or two. Stir-fry veggie strips and tofu in a hint of sesame oil. Or cook up spaghetti, peas, and chopped tomatoes, and top with a sprinkle of parmesan cheese.

Change the focus of the meal from a slab of meat to meat strips. Serve up beef or chicken fajitas: lightly marinated, grilled strips of meat assembled on a tortilla with cooked tomatoes, onions, and peppers. Or discover shish kabob: skewer lean meats or chunks of fish alongside fruit or vegetable chunks. Grill or broil, basting with jam or marmalade.

smart shopping

What doesn't go in the cart won't end up around your waist

When your kitchen is well-stocked with easy-to-prepare, nutritious foods, healthful eating is fun, easy, and interesting. The key is to put the right things in the shopping cart when you're in the grocery store.

Starting this week, buy a spice, fruit, vegetable, or grain you've never used before. Choose something that's easy to make, so you don't agonize over the preparation. For example, try artichoke hearts in a can (in water, not oil), wild rice, kiwis, or bagged spring salad mix. Stock up on fruit. It's loaded with vitamins, and it tastes so good. (Buy some fruit that's already cut up—yes, it's more expensive, but it's worth it if you eat that instead of a bag of chips.) You and your family are much more likely to reach for fruits like melons, pineapples, and kiwis when they are already peeled and ready to eat.

The next time you go shopping, buy staples that make healthful cooking quick, tasty, and easy. Include low-fat and low-sodium broths and marinades; couscous; all varieties of canned beans, chick peas, and lentils; canned tuna and salmon in water; chopped nuts; herbs, all-fruit spreads, fruit juices, yogurt, and vinegars to flavor your food without salt and fats; and raw veggies.

Buy fresh or frozen vegetables instead of canned, when possible, to reduce sodium, syrup, sauce, sugar, fats, butter, or other additives. (You can always spice things up yourself.) Pre-cut vegetables can simplify cooking and help vary your fare. (When was the last time you used okra, lima beans, cauliflower, butternut squash, mustard greens, or black-eyed peas? They're all available, trimmed and washed, in the freezer section.) Just open the bag and drop veggies in soup, tomato sauce, stir-frys, or stew.

Buy plenty of low- or no-fat plain yogurt to substitute for sour cream on potatoes, to add to rice and beans to give them a creamy texture, to be the base for fruit smoothies and vegetable dip, to add to mashed potatoes and pancake mix, and for much, much more.

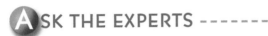

ASK THE EXPERTS

I buy the right foods, but then I don't eat them. When evening comes and I want a snack, I bypass the baby carrots and dig into the cookies. Any suggestions?

Don't buy the cookies. Or the ice cream, cupcakes, chips, cereal bars, or whatever it is that does you in. If you don't buy it, you won't have it in the house. Then you can't eat it. (Make sure you're not hungry when you go shopping, or you're apt to buy everything in sight.) If this idea makes you crazy, only buy single servings of snacks. You're less likely to scarf down half a container of ice cream if you buy frozen fruit bars or individually wrapped fudge pops. Or make the carrots a bit more inviting with a low-fat dip.

I'm confused. My brother tells me I'm no better off buying ground turkey or ground chicken to save on fat. And that wheat bread is nothing special, either. Is he right?

It depends on what you buy. Unless the label specifies ground *breast* meat or *white* meat, ground turkey or chicken can be loaded with fat. As for the wheat bread, your brother is right. Unless the label specifies *whole wheat* bread, you're probably eating white bread with molasses or caramel coloring.

EASE INTO IT

Write down the fruits and vegetables you ate yesterday. Did you reach five servings? Did you include sources of vitamins A and C? Map out what and when you can eat tomorrow to reach five servings of fruits and vegetables.

healthful cooking

Give your recipes a makeover

You don't need to ban your family's favorite foods in order to cook healthfully. Often, you just need to tweak your recipes a bit. Substitute healthier alternatives for saturated fats, use leaner meats and cheeses, and integrate fruits, vegetables, and whole grains.

Take your famous Sunday morning French toast, for example. Eliminate a few yolks in the egg mixture and swap vegetable oil spray for butter on the skillet and you erase lots of fat and cholesterol. Use whole grain bread instead of white to load up on fiber. The French toast will taste a lot like it did before—you may even like it better—and it will be much healthier for you.

Subtle changes in your cooking can mean significant changes to your waistline. Sauté or brown meats in non-stick skillets misted with vegetable oil. Sauté vegetables in a bit of broth, wine, or juice instead of oil or butter. Use broth instead of water and butter when cooking couscous or rice.

Roast, bake, broil, stir-fry, or grill meats and fish instead of frying in oil or butter. When you need to add fat, make it canola, olive, sunflower, safflower, or corn oil.

FITNESS FACTS

Using Your Noodle

You can swap lean ground turkey breast for ground beef, but if you can't bear the thought of ground turkey in your signature lasagna, replace just one layer of sausage or ground beef with a layer of roasted vegetable chunks. To further reduce fat, switch from whole milk ricotta and mozzarella cheese to low-fat. Grate cheese to spread it out and use less. To really turn the tables on fat, don't use ricotta at all. Instead, whirl low-fat cottage cheese in the blender and you end up with the same creamy consistency as ricotta and save hundreds of calories and dozens of grams of fat per serving.

Too Much of a Good Thing? No!

Want to make healthful cooking a snap? Prepare extra. But don't eat it immediately! Cooking rice with dinner? Make more than you need and use it for tomorrow's rice and bean salad lunch. Whipping up nutritious pancakes? Make extra for the freezer. When you're running late, simply pop a couple of pancakes in the microwave or toaster oven instead of grabbing a donut on the way to work. Cutting up carrots or trimming green beans for dinner? Fix a few more to snack on at work tomorrow. Roasting chicken or turkey? Plan for enough leftovers for tomorrow's lunch. Combine with salad greens, half an apple, a few dried cranberries and chopped almonds, and light honey-mustard salad dressing, and you have lunch in a flash. Making soup from scratch? Remove some broth and stick it in the freezer. When you want a yummy and healthy lunch in a jiffy, heat the frozen broth and add it to couscous and last night's vegetables. The options are endless.

smart snacking

*Put some
punch in
your crunch*

Many people manage to eat decently at meal time, only to be done in by the wrong snacks. A handful of chocolate kisses here, a bag of chips there, a cup or two or three of ice cream. Before you know it, the pounds pile on.

Instead of packing on the fat, snacks can be terrific tasty tools for boosting energy and filling out the day's nutrition needs. But what should you eat and when? How can you be sure to snack smart? First, snack at the right time. Remember the food diary you compiled in *Nutrition Basics*? If you're always famished at a certain time of day, eat a snack about 15 minutes before hunger pangs usually strike, so you don't inhale everything in sight.

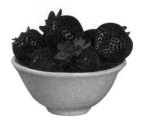

Choose something that fills in servings from the pyramid or has nutrients you might otherwise miss. A cup of strawberries, for example, takes care of two fruit servings and all the vitamin C you need for the day. A big handful of whole wheat pretzels fits the bill for a grain serving. A bowl of whole grain cereal with skim milk and half a banana satisfies some dairy, grain, and fruit requirements and is mighty filling and tasty, too.

If you have healthful snacks available at home and work you're less likely to reach for something unhealthy. Be proactive. Add good snacks like whole grain crackers, low-fat yogurt and cheese, fruit, and vegetable sticks to your shopping list. If you feel industrious, make bread or muffins with pumpkin, zucchini, corn, cranberry, banana, bran, apple, or blueberry filling. A slice of cheese and some fruit, or a handful of raisins and almonds, or dried fruits and cereal almost always do the trick. A baked potato with salsa works well, too.

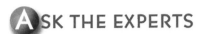

ASK THE EXPERTS

What if I want something substantial to tide me over for a while?

Aim for some combination of protein and carbohydrates. A bowl of vegetable bean soup could be perfect. Other examples: chopped fresh fruit over a half cup of cottage cheese, a hard-boiled egg with some carrot sticks on the side, an apple and a slice of cheddar cheese, or homemade trail mix (whole grain cereal, chopped dried fruits, and chopped nuts).

When I'm home in front of the TV, I crave crunchy. What can I try?

Air-popped light popcorn is an ideal choice. Spice it up with cinnamon, parmesan cheese, or chili powder. Other good crunchy choices include cereal; pretzels; carrots, peppers, cauliflower, snap peas, green beans, broccoli, or celery dipped in fat-free plain yogurt with herbs or Dijon mustard; a crisp apple; nuts mixed with raisins and cereal; or rice cakes.

Healthy-crunchy doesn't work for me. I crave cool and creamy. Any suggestions?

Sure. Low-fat or no-fat flavored yogurt is an excellent choice. Toss in a handful of granola cereal if you want a little more oomph in each bite. For a close-to-perfect snack, combine in the blender 1 cup of low- or no-fat plain yogurt; a handful of ice cubes; half a banana; 1/2 cup of berries, mango or cantaloupe; a teaspoon of maple syrup or honey; and a shake of cinnamon. Or skip the sweeteners and cinnamon and use a flavored yogurt, such as chocolate, peach, or mocha.

now what do I do?

Answers to common questions

Q I just can't bring myself to do another chore, and healthful cooking seems so burdensome. What can I do?

Spice up the process. Make cooking fun! Cook together with family members or your best friends. Put on your Andrea Boccelli CD, muster up a big batch of spaghetti sauce, vegetable chili, or chicken soup, and dance, play a board game, or just enjoy your time together while the sauce, chili, or soup simmers. (If you really want to make a healthy time of it, put on an exercise video and work out together while the food cooks!) Then split the batch into portions and put them in the freezer. You end up with healthy food and fun, quality time.

Q Should I make sure that whatever I buy is fat-free and cholesterol-free?

Not necessarily. Just because something is labeled fat-free or cholesterol-free doesn't mean it's the best option. The item might still pack a wallop in the calorie department and could be loaded with fillers instead of nutritious ingredients. Check the nutrition label (you learned how to read it in *Nutrition Basics*) and compare calories and nutrients between fat-free and regular items to determine the best choice.

Q I have a family of picky eaters. I don't see them embracing new foods just because of the health benefits. What should I do?

Give the family favorites a makeover. If your family likes spaghetti with meat sauce, add chopped vegetables to the sauce. Or skip the meat and add a can of tuna and some scallops to the tomato sauce. Even change the spaghetti to spaghetti squash. Similarly, change meat-and-potatoes to just potatoes. Take a baked potato from its shell and mix with low-fat cottage cheese or low- or non-fat plain yogurt. Top with chopped steamed veggies like broccoli or zucchini and finish off with salsa or tomato sauce. And don't be afraid to experiment with low-fat, low-calorie powdered butter substitutes. They work well in moist dishes such as mashed potatoes or on steamed vegetables.

BOOKS

Food Shopping Counter, Annette Natow and JoAnn Heslin
Strategies for healthful shopping, label-reading tips; calories, fat, sodium, carbs, and fiber counts for more than 20,000 foods.

The Unofficial Guide to Smart Nutrition, Ross Hume Hall, Ph.D.
A comprehensive, anti-establishment look at what's really in food; the ABCs of supplements and the relationship between nutrition and disease.

WEB SITES

www.nal.usda.gov
The USDA's Food and Nutrition Information Center. Lists dietary guidelines, the Food Guide Pyramid, a nutrient database, links to other sites and more. From here, visit the Interactive Healthy Eating Index at **www. usda.gov/cnpp**, which shows how well your diet meets the dietary guidelines and the Food Guide Pyramid, and provides recipes and tips for healthy, inexpensive meals.

www.deliciousdecisions.org
Recipes, supermarket tips, and advice on how to get fit and eat out, from the American Heart Association.

www.ediets.com
Offers custom-tailored online weight-loss programs, for a monthly fee. Subscription includes weekly menus, recipes, and grocery lists, along with information on nutrition, exercise, motivation, and support.

www.mealsforyou.com
Thousands of recipes, meal plans, and shopping lists, including recipes categorized by the nutritional content of the foods.

ORGANIZATIONS

The American Dietetic Association
(800) 366-1655
www.eatright.org
To find a dietitian near you; get daily nutrition, fitness, and healthy lifestyle tips; learn the latest in nutrition news.

PUBLICATIONS

Tufts University Diet and Nutrition Letter
(800) 274-7581
www.healthletter.tufts.edu
Up-to-date nutrition news, strategy, and advice. The Web site includes sample articles and subscription information.

The New Dietary Guidelines for Americans
For a copy, send 50 cents to Consumer Information Center, Department 378-C, Pueblo, CO 81009. The guidelines are free on the Internet at **www.usda.gov/cnpp**.

4

weight management

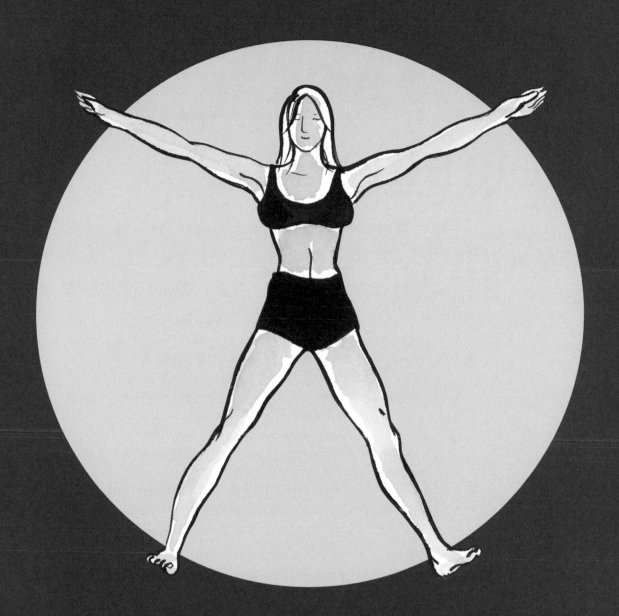

Managing and maintaining your weight
is an important aspect of living a long,
healthy life. Learn what your healthy
weight range should be and how
you can get there—safely.

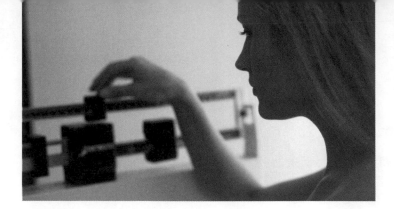

weighing in

What do you have to lose?

How do you know if you need to trim down? You should consider losing weight if:

- Your BMI is 25 or above. (A BMI of 30 or greater is considered obese.)
- Your weight exceeds the "healthy" range on the chart on the right. (Note: Someone with a lot of muscle may be above the "healthy" range and may not need to trim down.)
- You have excess weight around your middle. (Go back to *Shaping Up*, where you calculated your waist-to-hip ratio.) If you're an "apple" (your body fat is concentrated around your abdomen), you have a higher risk of weight-related health problems than if you're a "pear" (you carry your fat on your buttocks and thighs). Males whose waist-to-hip ratio is .95 or higher and females whose ratio exceeds .80 are at the greatest risk.
- You suffer from weight-related medical problems such as diabetes, high blood pressure, high cholesterol, or joint problems.

FITNESS FACTS: DO YOU NEED TO GAIN WEIGHT?

If you're below the healthy weight range or if you have a BMI of less than 18.5, you are considered underweight. Being underweight is linked to heart problems and lower resistance to infection.

If you're not sure whether or not your weight is right for you, see your physician or a registered dietitian.

Check with your physician to find out if your low weight is caused by a medical problem.

Why Lose Weight?

There are tons of reasons. Among them, excess weight hikes your risk of heart disease, stroke, Type 2 diabetes, high blood pressure and cholesterol, certain cancers, arthritis, gallbladder disease, lung problems, gynecological problems, sleep apnea, gallstones, and gout. The more body fat you have, the harder your lungs, heart, and skeleton have to work. A person who is 40 percent overweight is twice as likely to die prematurely as someone of average weight. Being overweight can also take an emotional toll: Heavy people may face discrimination, suffer depression, and feel shame—as slimness is equated with attractiveness in American culture.

The heavier you are, the harder it is to be physically active—even to perform everyday activities. This feeds the cycle of excess weight: The less active you are, the fewer calories you burn and the less able you are to lose weight.

Good news: If you're overweight, trimming your weight by as little as 5 or 10 percent can slice your risk of weight-related health problems. And that's definitely worth the effort!

Note: If you take medications, have health problems, smoke, aim to lose more than 15 or 20 pounds, or are over 50 years old (or over 35 and sedentary) see your physician before starting any weight-loss regimen.

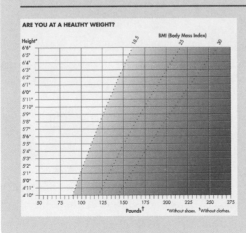

ARE YOU AT A HEALTHY WEIGHT?

going for the goal

*The shape
of things
to come*

You can shed pounds without following complicated plans, eating frozen or liquid meals, craving your favorite foods, or shelling out your hard-earned money. But if you want to keep off extra pounds for good, traveling warp speed isn't the best way to get there. (After all, it took time to put on the weight.)

Instead, climb aboard a slow, steady train. There will be a few bumps. You may have to adjust your itinerary. But you'll get to your destination and still enjoy the foods you like.

First, figure out your motivation to take the trip. Why do you want to lose or maintain weight? If your motivation is to wear that size 8 dress or that slim-cut suit to your high school reunion next month, you may not make it for the long haul because you won't have a reason to keep the weight off in the future.

On the other hand, if your motivation is to be healthy and feel good about yourself, you're more likely to adopt eating and exercise habits that will keep the weight off.

FITNESS FACTS

The Buddy System

Why travel alone? Having a support system can make your weight-control efforts easier and help you stay on track. The right person can lend an ear when the going gets tough, pepper you with compliments, and cheer you on. But beware of saboteurs: they undermine your efforts, urging you to eat foods you're trying to avoid, insisting you've lost enough weight, dispensing unsolicited advice about what you should and shouldn't eat. Think of someone who has been supportive of you in the past and even someone who is on a similar quest. Ask him or her to be your supporter. Explain your weight-management plan, why it's important to you, and what you're looking for in a support person. If you prefer, search online for support groups or start your own. Join a group that offers support, such as Overeaters Anonymous (for compulsive eaters) or TOPS (Take Off Pounds Sensibly). Or seek support from a registered dietitian or another nutrition professional.

SETTING GOALS

Now you know why you're on the journey. It's time to set realistic goals. Often people set themselves up to fail by striving for goals that are impossible to achieve, such as dropping 35 pounds in two months or swearing off a favorite food. Then, when they don't meet these unrealistic goals—and they probably won't—they're apt to feel defeated and give up.

Instead, shoot for goals that are:

Realistic. Aim to lose one or two pounds—even half a pound—a week. Your desirable weight should be your healthy weight—not a weight you haven't seen since you were 12! Strive to cut back on unhealthful foods, not necessarily to eliminate them.

Short-term. For example, say you want to lose 5 to 10 percent of your weight in a year (a reasonable goal) and to keep it off. Aim to shed five pounds and to walk half a mile a day by the end of the month. Once you reach that short-term goal, your success will motivate you to achieve the next goal.

Each time you meet a mini-goal, **reward yourself.** Go to a movie, buy the latest CD, treat yourself to flowers, splurge on a new pair of shoes, take a little trip. The reward that awaits you will inspire you to meet your next goal. Expect success!

And keep writing in your **food diary.** Studies show that people who monitor what they eat and drink are more successful at weight management. Note what you eat and drink, your hunger level, and what you were feeling when you ate. Then keep track of your weight. Use your diary to discover what works and what doesn't, then fine-tune.

removing
the obstacles

*Don't let
your triggers
trip you up*

Take a look at your food-diary entries. Do you eat when you're not hungry? Do you chow down when you're bored, lonely, or stressed? Do you clean your plate as your parents taught you? Do you nibble when you watch the news? Do you finish off the fries on little Frankie's plate? If you're like most people, you do some (or all!) of these things. Certain triggers can weaken your resolve and lead to overeating. But if you manage these triggers and learn to eat when you're hungry and stop when you're satisfied, you'll be in control of your eating. Here are some helpful tips to keep you on track:

If you eat to cope with your emotions, find alternatives: Call a friend, take a walk (this also burns calories!), meditate, take a few deep breaths, garden, or read a book. Try to recognize the signs of hunger, satisfaction, and fullness. Learn to tell the difference between these and an emotional urge to eat. When you feel that emotional urge, set a timer for 15 minutes and do something else. The urge is likely to pass.

Brush your teeth if you feel like eating when you're not hungry: the taste of the toothpaste may kill the urge.

If you eat while watching TV, you can lose track of what's going into your mouth. Instead of eating, busy your hands with a hobby.

If you have a habit of grabbing the goodies next to the coffee pot at work, have a colleague get your coffee for you until your will power is stronger.

To avoid eating leftover food from plates when you clean up after a meal, immediately scrape the food into the trash.

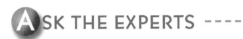SK THE EXPERTS

I really want to eat when I'm stressed. What if I can't resist the urge?
Choose foods that won't sabotage your efforts. When you're angry or tense, try eating crunchy foods like carrots, pretzels, apples, or popcorn (hold the butter). Soft, creamy foods such as low- or non-fat yogurt may help if you seek comfort. When you're not in that stressful moment, write a list of things you can do when you get that urge, such as taking a walk or pushing your kids on the swings. Post it in a visible place, so you'll have alternatives when you go to reach for the ice cream.

How often should I weigh myself?
Definitely not every day. Your weight fluctuates from day to day, so you may get discouraged if the number on the scale doesn't change, or is higher. Weigh in once a week—or every two weeks—and you'll get extra motivation by seeing that lower number. Wear clothes of the same weight (or none at all) each time you weigh in, and step on the scale at the same time of day. If you can, don't weigh yourself at all. Judge your progress by how you feel, how your clothes fit, and what you're able to do.

Now you know where you're headed. How will you get there? Take the route that fits your needs, your likes and dislikes, your budget, and your schedule.

slimming secrets

Finding your ticket to a healthy weight

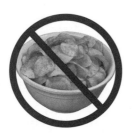

Here's the secret to weight management (drum roll, please): Managing your weight is simply a matter of managing calories. To lose weight, either scale back the calories you consume or boost the calories you burn. (It's best to do both.) To maintain your weight, balance the calories you take in and expend.

Chances are, if you're overweight, you consume more calories than you need. To lose one pound, you must burn 3,500 more calories than you take in. Trim your daily calories by just 250—say, your morning donut and that tablespoon of mayonnaise on your sandwich—and you'll lose 26 pounds in a year. Walk 30 minutes, burning 160 calories, five times a week, and you'll drop another 12 pounds. Lower your daily calories by 500—cut out the chips with lunch and the evening cup of ice cream, for example—and you'll lose a pound in a week. That's 52 pounds in a year!

The Food Guide Pyramid and the Dietary Guidelines are your tour guides. From the pyramid, choose lower calorie foods within each group, opt for the low end of the recommended servings, and you'll take in about 1,600 calories a day.

• Don't consume fewer than 1,200 calories a day if you're a woman or 1,600 if you're a man, or you may not get enough nutrients and may shift your body into starvation mode. This is when your body conserves energy by slowing the rate you burn calories.

• Trim calories by eating less fat, as each gram of fat contains 9 calories, compared to 4 calories for carbs and proteins. When you reduce your fat intake, you can eat more food for the same number of calories! This frees up room for healthful, lower-calorie foods like whole grains, fruits, and vegetables.

• Limit fat to about 30 percent of your daily calories—and saturated fats to less than 10 percent—to help your heart and your waistline. Don't let your fat intake drop below 10 percent, though: fat is essential to your body.

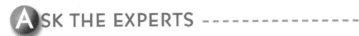

ASK THE EXPERTS

Do I have to give up my favorite snack, cheesecake with a tall glass of milk?

Change one small thing at a time and build on your success. For example, you don't have to switch from whole milk to skim in one fell swoop. Instead, drop to 2 percent, then to 1 percent. Reduce the two pats of butter on your baked potato to one. Next, replace one red-meat meal with a fish meal.

Eat foods you enjoy. If you deprive yourself of cheesecake, you may crave it sooner or later. You'll give in to the craving and eat half a cake, or worse, give up your shape-up effort. The key is to have the cheesecake less often—once a month, say—and to eat smaller portions of it.

Whenever I try to lose weight, I blow it and then give up. Any suggestions?

Swear off "should," "never," and "always" from your vocabulary. No food is forbidden. No food is "bad." Don't beat yourself up if you slip off your new eating style. Shake off the guilt and avoid negative talk. Talk to yourself as you'd talk to a friend. Just get back on track. Perseverance, not perfection, is the key.

Will exercise help me lose weight?

Absolutely. While changing your eating habits does the most to trim pounds, exercising regularly is like having the wind at your back as you sail. It will get you to your weight destination more quickly.

practical diet tips

Easy-to-follow pointers to ensure success

Here is your blueprint for success—simple changes you can make to help reach your desirable weight. Remember, what counts is what you eat over several days, not just at one meal.

Choose fruits, vegetables, and whole grains as the bulk of your meals. They're high in fiber and low in fat and calories.

Hold the butter, creamy sauces, and foods packed in sugar. Cut back on baked goods, sugary cereals, chips loaded with fat, processed meats (bacon, hot dogs, salami), and creamy soups.

Choose lean meats and fish. Eat meat and dairy products as smaller portions of your meals. Trim the fat from meat and remove the skin from poultry. Enjoy nuts on occasion.

Go for whole fruit, rather than fruit juice. (An orange, for example, is more filling than a cup of orange juice.) Or dilute juice with water.

Limit your alcohol: 12 ounces of beer pack 150 calories and 5 ounces of wine contain 100 calories.

Refrigerate a can of soup a few hours before you open it. The fat will rise to the top, where you can skim it.

Eat low-fat or non-fat dairy products.

Use reduced-calorie salad dressings.

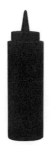

Spice up foods with ketchup, mustard, barbecue sauce, or salsa instead of mayo, sour cream, or butter.

Instead of high-sugar soda, drink seltzer water with lemon.

Eat protein at every meal to keep your hunger in check.

Eat three meals a day, or six smaller meals—whichever works best.

Keep lower calorie snacks (apples, carrot sticks, air-popped popcorn, raisins) on hand for when hunger strikes.

Drink lots of water throughout the day. Your body needs it.

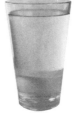

Find delicious, low-calorie recipes in cookbooks, magazines, and on the Internet.

Plan your meals and snacks for the week, and make a list before you shop. Stick to what's on your list, and don't shop on an empty stomach when impulsive buying can occur. Don't buy foods you're trying not to eat, such as chips.

Instead of frying foods, bake, broil, stew, steam, grill, or roast them.

Eat sitting down—only at the kitchen or dining room table. And don't eat out of packages, as it's easy to lose track of how much you eat.

Use a smaller plate so it looks like there's more on it.

If you get hungry before your usual mealtime, eat some of your meal earlier and the rest at your regular mealtime. Better yet, move up your mealtime.

Start meals with the lowest-calorie foods, such as vegetables and soup, and accompany them with water, seltzer, or tea. By the time you get to the highest-calorie part of your meal (the meat, for example), you may be full enough to eat less of it.

Eat slowly. It takes about 20 minutes for your brain to receive the message that you've had enough food. If you eat quickly, you're likely to overeat before you realize you've had enough.

dieting downsides

Why diets don't work for the long haul

Does this sound familiar? You diet, you lose weight, you put it back on. You diet, you lose weight, you put it back on. If so, you're not alone. As you read this, about half of all women and 25 percent of men in the United States are on diets. Only a fraction—about 5 percent—maintain the loss after a year, and many will regain more than they lost!

The pounds may melt away when you diet, especially in the beginning, when you lose mostly water, not body fat. But most diets don't work for the long haul.

Why? Most diets tend to focus on the short-term. They often restrict food choices and limit you to very small portions and very few calories. No wonder you lose weight!

These severe restrictions are impossible to maintain for the long haul. After all, how long can you consume cabbage soup or eat miniscule portions? After a while, a few things can happen. You may fear food, thinking of it as "bad." You may obsess about food: It becomes the forbidden fruit. You may crave forbidden foods so much that you break the diet, overeat, or binge. Then you feel like a failure. And when you return to your former eating habits—which inevitably happens if the diet doesn't teach you how to eat healthfully—the pounds sneak back on.

Restrictive diets may rob you of the nutrients your body needs, depleting your energy and hiking your risk of nutrient deficiencies. In addition, severe diets can cause you to lose not just body fat, but also an excessive amount of muscle tissue.

Dieting is an option if you want to drop a few pounds before your brother's wedding. Just don't expect to keep it off when the party's over. A diet that doesn't teach you new eating and exercise habits is plugging your flat tire with a wad of gum. It may work for a short while, but before long, you're back where you started.

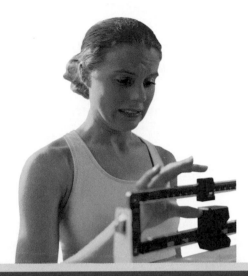

Buyer (and Dieter) Beware

Steer clear of diets or products that:

- Pronounce certain foods as good or bad ("Watermelon will burn the fat.")
- Use someone else's results to predict yours ("Dana lost 70 pounds in 70 days.")
- Promise quick and effortless results ("Wear the magic weight-loss bracelet and lose 10 pounds.")
- Sound too good to be true ("Eat whatever you want and lose weight.")
- Claim to take pounds off for good ("Permanent weight loss guaranteed.")
- Are based on one study or studies that haven't been reviewed by peers
- Are refuted by reputable organizations

sizing up popular diets

From low-carb to high protein, fad diets abound

They're everywhere you turn, from Oprah to the bookstores, from the Internet to your favorite magazine. Most likely, at least several people in your circle (even you) have tried a diet that's all the rage. Chances are, they lost weight. Unfortunately, they also probably gained it back.

Sorting through the diets can get mighty confusing: Each author claims his or her diet is the answer. One diet contradicts another. They all claim to be based on scientific evidence. Even so, it's tempting to simply pick up one of the popular diet books and follow the plan. But before you do, know this: The reason people gain weight is that they consume more calories than they use. It doesn't matter whether those extra calories come from carbs, protein, or fat.

HERE'S THE LOWDOWN ON SOME POPULAR DIETS:

High protein, low-carbohydrate diets

Americans are heavier than ever because they eat too many carbohydrates, or so claim these diet creators. They say that eating too many carbohydrates raises your blood sugar and causes your body to produce too much **insulin**, a hormone that delivers glucose to your cells. They claim that this is what causes hunger and weight gain. The theory is that a low-carbohydrate diet results in less insulin to draw on, so your body burns its fat reserves for energy, which makes you lose weight.

The truth is that any rapid drop in weight on these diets is most likely the loss of water. You also may lose weight because the diets are low in calories, because protein and fat are filling, and because you have less of an appetite. But at what price? Carbohydrates are your body's preferred source of energy. When they aren't available, your body turns to fats for energy and **ketones** (by-products of breaking down fat) build up in your blood. This causes **ketosis** (an excess of ketones), which curbs hunger but also stresses your kidneys and can cause fatigue, nausea, dehydration, bad breath, an increased risk for kidney disease, and gout. Ketosis can be dangerous for people who are diabetic or pregnant.

Low-carb diets **contradict** the Dietary Guidelines and the Food Guide Pyramid, which recommend that a majority of your daily calories come from carbs, and about 30 percent from fat. Some of these diets are high in fat, which ups your risk of heart disease and certain cancers, particularly if they're high in **saturated fat** (fat from animal products, such as butter or meat). And if your protein sources are mainly from animals, you ingest a lot of dietary cholesterol, which boosts your risk of heart disease. Diets that restrict carbs such as fruits, vegetables, and whole grains rob you of certain vitamins and minerals, as well as fiber and phytochemicals (substances in plants that fight disease).

For some people, eating a diet very high in carbohydrates can hike their insulin and triglyceride levels. They may need to eat a bit less carbohydrate and more fat. But there's no scientific evidence that high insulin levels stimulate your appetite or make you store more fat and gain weight; or that very low-carb diets are any more effective than other reduced-calorie diets.

High-fiber, low-fat diets

Some diets tout eating more **fiber** to help you lose weight. Fiber is filling and takes longer to chew, so you may consume fewer calories. Moreover, fiber slows the absorption of foods, delaying hunger. High-fiber foods—fruits, veggies, and whole grains—are healthful, but eating too much fiber can cause diarrhea, gassiness, bloating, and abdominal pain.

diet drinks and pills

Is there a magic bullet?

With many people looking for a magic bullet, options abound in the weight-loss world. Most have limited effectiveness—and some are downright dangerous.

Over-the-counter meal replacements: Pop a can. Pour powder in a glass and add liquid. Tear into a bar. What could be easier? By replacing two meals with liquid drinks or packaged foods, products aim to restrict total calorie intake. Each meal replacement packs only about 200 calories, so you'll need tons of willpower not to scarf down everything in sight for your third meal. The products provide nutrients, but lack the phytochemicals you get from fruits and vegetables. Ingesting so few calories can put your body in starvation mode, making you burn calories more slowly. That's the last thing you want to happen! You may lose weight on these products, but you shouldn't expect to keep it off without changing your lifestyle.

Over-the-counter drugs: There's no shortage of over-the-counter weight-loss drugs and herbal preparations on the market. For most, little scientific evidence exists on their safety and effectiveness. Many, such as Acutrim and Dexatrim, contain phenylpropanolamine (PPA), a stimulant and an appetite suppressant that may help you lose a little weight. It can, however, cause serious side effects if you exceed the recommended dosage. Other over-the-counter medications contain caffeine, which is a stimulant and a diuretic. These products only help you lose water. Stay clear of chromium picolinate (which may cause kidney failure and is not recommended for weight loss), and the laxative senna (which only causes water loss and may produce side effects). Ephedrine (the ingredient in ephedra, known as ma huang), is an amphetamine-like substance that suppresses appetite, and can cause serious, sometimes fatal, side effects. It is not recommended for weight loss.

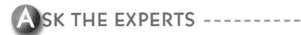

ASK THE EXPERTS

I should lose about 40 pounds. Are there any prescription weight-loss drugs that would help?

This is an option for people whose obesity or extra weight poses a serious health risk. Drugs such as **sibutramine** (Meridia) suppress appetite by altering brain chemicals. Others, such as **orlistat** (Xenical), inhibit the absorption of fat. Weight-loss medications do not result in permanent weight loss and are best used as part of a weight-management program that stresses changes in eating and physical activity. As with any medication, beware of potential side effects. Talk with your physician about this option.

What about products like rubber clothes that promise to take off weight ? Do they work?

You might as well throw your dollars down the drain. Most of these "wonder" products are fraudulent and some are even dangerous. Among the gadgets that won't melt away pounds are earrings, patches, appetite-suppressing eyeglasses, creams, and electrical muscle stimulators. Wearing special rubber or nylon garments causes water loss from sweating, not loss of body fat.

I'm sick of being so heavy. Should I consider surgery?

That depends. If you're more than 100 pounds overweight and have significant medical problems associated with your weight, you may want to discuss **gastric** (stomach) **stapling** and **gastric bypass** with your physician. These procedures reduce the size of your stomach, limiting how much food you can eat and absorb. **Liposuction**, surgery to remove fat using a suction pump, is an option for people of normal weight who have pockets of excess fat in certain areas. **Abdominoplasty** ("tummy tuck") removes excess skin and fat, and tightens muscles in the abdominal area. All of these procedures carry medical risks.

joining a program

Weight-loss programs put your money where your mouth is

If you like the camaraderie of a group or the structure of a diet plan or if you need professional support or medical supervision, joining a weight-loss program might be the ticket.

HERE'S THE SKINNY ON WHAT SOME COMMERCIAL WEIGHT-LOSS PROGRAMS SERVE UP!

Jenny Craig uses prepackaged low-calorie meals and snacks, followed by a transition to regular foods halfway through your weight loss. The program stresses lifestyle change, including exercise, diet, and stress management. Trained employees staff the program. You'll shell out $200 to $350 to join, and prepackaged foods run about $70 to $85 per week. Weekly individual counseling is included, and a maintenance program is available. Prepackaged foods are convenient, but can get tedious.

The Solution is based on the premise that you can achieve permanent weight loss by getting to the root of being overweight and by making lifestyle, mind, and body changes. Staffed by registered dietitians and mental health professionals, The Solution provides counseling and education on healthful eating, and promotes exercise. Courses (including via telephone) cost $400 and up, plus materials. This program may be too abstract for some.

Weight Watchers assigns points to foods according to their fat, fiber, and calorie content, and allows you a certain number of points, based on your weight. As long as you stay within your points, you can choose whatever foods or beverages you like. Weekly group meetings, staffed by trained employees, cover lifestyle change, including exercise. The

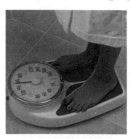

program is relatively inexpensive because you buy your own foods: about $15 to join, and $10 to $12 a week for the weight-loss phase and maintenance. (Weight Watchers foods are available.) The downsides are you may not like keeping track of points, and it is possible to stay within your points and choose foods that are not nutritious.

Clinical Programs such as Optifast and Health Management Resources (HMR) operate in hospitals, clinics, and physicians' offices. Most often, they replace meals with very-low-calorie formulas and prepackaged foods, and are geared to the seriously overweight. Typically, the programs include a weight-loss phase of 10 to 20 weeks, a transition back to normal food, and maintenance. In addition to providing rapid weight loss, they emphasize healthful eating and exercise habits. Supervised by physicians, they are often staffed by registered nurses, dietitians, and exercise experts. Very-low-calorie diets may cause side effects, and at a cost of up to $3,000, these programs can take a bite out of your wallet.

FITNESS FACTS

Check Out the Program

If you are considering a weight-loss program, make sure it:

- Aims for weight loss of 1 to 2 pounds a week, unless your medical condition warrants rapid weight loss
- Provides counseling on how to change eating and physical activity habits
- Provides adequate amounts of nutrients
- Is designed and supervised by qualified health professionals, such as registered dietitians, nutritionists, doctors, nurses, psychologists, and exercise physiologists
- Takes into account the kinds of food you like and dislike

Before you sign on the dotted line, ask:

- How much does the program cost, including meal replacements, foods, supplements, membership, weekly fees, maintenance, and counseling? Are costs covered by health insurance or employers? What is the payment schedule? Do you refund money if clients drop out of the program?
- What is your clients' long-term success in maintaining their weight loss?
- What are the health risks of the program?
- What data do you have indicating that the program works?
- What are the credentials of the professional staff?
- Does the program have a maintenance program to help clients keep off weight?
- What percentage of your clients complete the program?
- What problems or side effects do your clients experience? What percentage of your clients experience them?

keeping it off

How to make your new weight stick

Congratulations! You've arrived at your weight destination. You like it here and want to stay—for a lifetime. How do you stay put?

Maintaining your weight—staying within 3 to 5 pounds of your desirable weight—can be as challenging as reaching that weight. The key, as with losing weight, is striking a balance between the calories you take in and the calories you expend.

Expect fluctuations of a few pounds. The amount of salt in the foods you eat, variations in food intake and elimination, how much you exercise and, if you're a woman, water retention around the time of menstruation, all affect your day-to-day weight.

Time to experiment. Try adding 200 calories or so to your daily diet. If you don't gain weight, stay there. If you're still losing weight at your new calorie level, add another 200 calories each day.

What if your weight inches up beyond those 3 to 5 pounds? First, check your food diary and your fitness log. Have you stopped exercising because of illness or bad weather or just *because*? Have you changed your eating habits? Use these tools to pinpoint problem areas, and make adjustments in what you eat and in your physical activity to get back on track. Write down what you like about your new weight (how you feel and look, for example) to motivate you to stick to your new lifestyle.

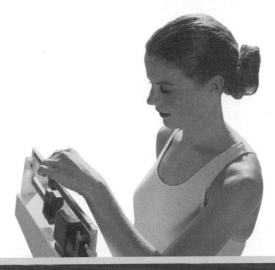

I wanted to lose 15 pounds, so I went on a diet. I had to make sure I ate exact amounts of protein and fat for two meals a day, and could only have carbs at one meal. I lost 5 pounds—and I was miserable. I couldn't eat what I wanted, when I wanted. I hated the structure of the diet, so I went off it and put the weight right back on. Then someone showed me the Food Guide Pyramid and I've been following it and watching what I eat. I stopped having soda every afternoon, use mustard instead of mayo, and put skim milk in my cappuccino. I even treat myself to my favorite food—fudge—once in a while. I joined a gym and work out four times a week. I don't feel deprived, I've already lost 9 pounds in two months, and best of all, I feel great! I think I can eat like this for good.

— Jennifer M., Dayton, Ohio

now what do I do?

Answers to common questions

Q I have ugly cellulite on my thighs. Will those products on the market help me get rid of it?

Sorry, but there's no quick fix to banish cellulite. Cellulite is normal body fat under your skin. When the fat thickens, connective tissue that holds fat in place shows through, looking lumpy. If you lose weight, the lumpiness may disappear, but no amount of creams or other "miracle" products will do the trick.

Q I know I should eat slowly, but it's hard for me. Any suggestions?

Sure. Try to make your meals last at least 20 minutes. Chew slowly and count to 10 before you take your next bite. A few more ideas for putting the brakes on: Listen to slow music while you eat, swallow before you take the next bite, stop eating once or twice during a meal for a minute or two, hold your fork in the hand you normally don't use, put your utensils down between bites, or use chopsticks!

Q I've been stuck at one weight for several weeks, but I still want to lose a few more pounds. Any suggestions?

Sounds like you've reached a plateau, the place on your journey where your weight stalls. This is normal. As you lose weight, your body becomes more efficient at using energy. Also, because you now weigh less, your body requires fewer calories. To get your weight loss out of neutral, tweak things a bit. Boost your metabolism by working out longer, harder, or more often: Walk a little faster, add 10 minutes to your bike rides, stop taking the elevator, and climb the stairs.

Q Should I count calories?

If you're up for it. Go back and calculate how many calories you'd need at your desirable weight. Shoot for eating at that level. (You will find calorie and nutrient contents for various foods on package labels, in books, and on Web sites such as www.nal.usda.gov.)

BOOKS

Eating Thin for Life: Food Secrets and Recipes From People Who Have Lost Weight and Kept It Off, Anne M. Fletcher, M.S., R.D.
How to control cravings, eat what you want, and stay motivated; plus recipes and menus.

The 9 Truths About Weight Loss: The No-Tricks, No-Nonsense Plan for Lifelong Weight Control, Daniel S. Kirschenbaum, Ph.D.
How to lose weight and keep it off by satisfying hunger, managing stress, and exercising. Endorsed by the American Council on Exercise.

The Solution, Laurel Mellin, M.A., R.D.
A six-step plan addressing the psychological, physical, and lifestyle causes of weight problems; how to maintain a healthy diet and an exercise program.

ORGANIZATIONS AND PROGRAMS

Health Management Resources
(800) 418-1367
www.yourbetterhealth.com
Weight-loss program offered in hospitals and medical centers providing low-calorie meals and snacks along with group meetings.

Jenny Craig
(800) 815-3669 **www.jennycraig.com**
Commercial weight-loss program with prepackaged foods that offers support and promotes lifestyle changes.

Optifast
(800) 662-2540 **www.optifast.com**
A medical weight-management program overseen by physicians, registered dietitians, and counselors that treats obesity with lifestyle modification and a calorie-controlled liquid nutritional formula.

TOPS (Take Off Pounds Sensibly)
(800) 932-8677 **www.tops.org**
An organization providing support, encouragement, and education to make healthy, permanent lifestyle changes. Membership includes weekly meetings and a magazine.

Weight Control Information Network
(877) 946-4627 **www.niddk.nih.gov/health /nutrit/win.htm**
A service of the National Institute of Health that provides information on obesity, weight control, and nutrition.

Weight Watchers International
(800) 651-6000
www.weightwatchers.com
Commercial weight-loss program offering eating program, support, and education on making lifestyle changes.

fitness that fits

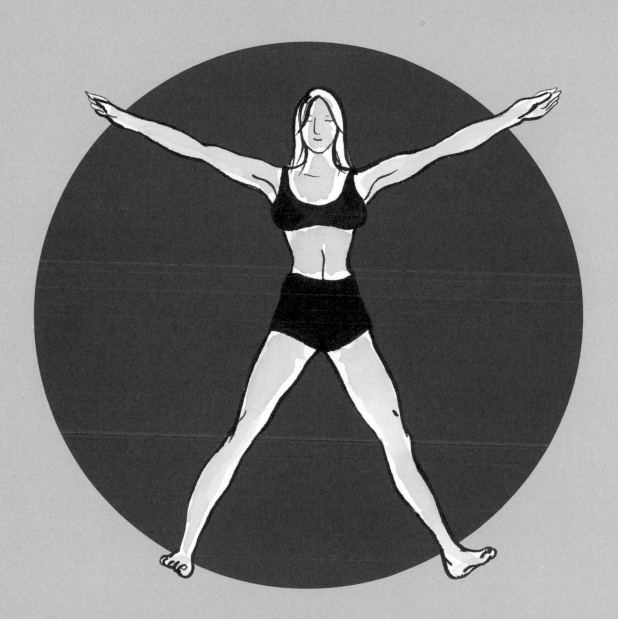

Exercise—it's the gift that keeps on giving.
That's because it continues to benefit you
long after you've hung up your sweats. Read
on and learn how to make it work for you.

basking in benefits

*Elements
of exercise*

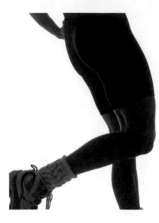

Raise your hand if you want to live longer with less stress, disease, and weight. Who doesn't want more energy, better health, and improved self-esteem? Now raise your other hand, twist and turn and jump around a little because if you want these benefits, you have to move your body. Go dancing, join a bowling league, play with the kids. It doesn't matter what physical activity you pick as long as you get your body in motion. And believe it or not, you'll feel great after working out.

Combined with healthy eating, physical activity clears the path to good fitness. In fact, exercising ranks right up there with quitting smoking in terms of lowering the risk of premature death.

In particular, exercise:
- increases flexibility and balance
- enhances the immune system
- heightens mental vigor
- boosts your energy and sense of well-being
- reduces the risk of heart attack

Exercise also reduces the risk of high blood pressure, colon cancer, adult onset diabetes, and physical injuries. It lowers bad cholesterol (LDL) levels and relieves anxiety.

Even if you haven't exercised in years—or if you never have—you can start benefiting today. It doesn't matter if you're 25 or 65. Studies show that when octogenarians start exercising with weights, they improve their strength, balance, and fitness. Some are even able to put their canes in storage and walk on their own.

HOT OFF THE BURNER

Exercise not only feels good, it burns calories. That helps you lose weight and keep it off. The more vigorously you exercise and the longer you do it, the more calories you burn. The heavier you are, the more you burn. Here's a snapshot:

CALORIES BURNED PER MINUTE IF YOU'RE:	120 LBS.	140 LBS.	160 LBS.	180 LBS.
ACTIVITY				
Basketball	7.5	8.8	10.0	11.3
Bowling	1.2	1.4	1.6	1.9
Boxing	8.1	9.5	10.9	12.3
Cycling (10 mph)	5.5	6.4	7.3	8.2
Dancing (aerobic)	7.4	8.6	9.8	11.1
Dancing (social)	2.9	3.3	3.7	4.2
Gardening	5.0	5.9	6.7	7.5
Golf (pull/carry clubs)	4.6	5.4	6.2	7.0
Golf (with cart)	2.1	2.5	2.8	3.2
Hiking	4.5	5.2	6.0	6.7
Jogging	9.3	10.8	12.4	13.9
Jumping rope	9.1	10.6	12.1	13.6
Running	11.4	13.2	15.1	17.0
Sitting	1.2	1.3	1.5	1.7
Skating (in-line)	5.9	7.4	8.5	9.5
Skiing (cross country)	7.5	8.8	10.0	11.3
Skiing (water and downhill)	5.7	6.6	7.6	8.5
Swimming (crawl, moderate pace)	7.8	9.0	10.3	11.6
Tennis	6.0	6.9	7.9	8.9
Walking (brisk)	6.5	7.6	8.7	9.7
Weight Training	6.6	7.6	8.7	9.8
Water Aerobics	3.6	4.2	4.8	5.5

Intensity changes things, too. A 150-pound person cycling at 12 miles per hour burns 9.5 calories a minute, and 14.2 calories a minute at 18 mph. The same person burns 4 calories a minute while walking a 20-minute mile, and 6.8 calories a minute while walking a 15-minute mile over hills.

Note: Before starting any exercise program, be sure to consult a physician.

getting physical

*Giving
your body
the workout
it needs*

If you're going to turn your body into a lean mean fit machine, you need to service it like a car. To keep your car not only humming and purring but able to merge on the highway in a hurry, you need to take care of all of it. You can't just wax the body and get new tires every now and then. While that takes care of cosmetics, it leaves the engine wanting and predisposed to failure. Same goes for your body. No matter what you do to keep up outside appearances, you need to work your entire body to get fit. As you read in *Shaping up*, you have to address all these aspects: cardiorespiratory fitness, muscle strength, flexibility, and body composition.

Cardiorespiratory, or **aerobic, fitness** is your body's ability to use oxygen to produce energy. **Aerobic exercise** is continuous and rhythmic physical motion using your large muscle groups. It challenges your circulatory and respiratory systems, keeping your heart pumping at an elevated, steady rate for an extended period. Aerobic exercises make your heart stronger and more efficient. They also help you maintain or lose weight.

Aerobic fitness is what gives you the energy to do an activity for a prolonged period: like walking two miles or swimming 10 laps. **Anaerobic fitness**, on the other hand, is how well your body draws stored energy that doesn't require oxygen. It's what you use for short bursts of activity, like running to catch a train. Regular aerobic exercise helps increase your anaerobic fitness.

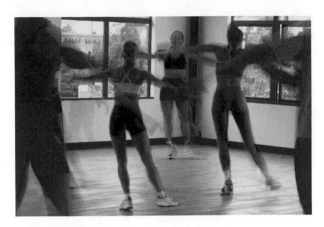

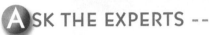

ASK THE EXPERTS

Can't I just do aerobics and get fit?

Sorry, while aerobic exercise is terrific for you and will help manage your weight, you'll need other components to get fit. You need to work your muscle strength (the amount of force your muscles can exert) and muscle endurance (your muscles' ability to exert force repeatedly). Although aerobic exercise will improve the tone and endurance of muscles, the muscles will get stronger only with strength training.

What else do I have to do?

All that pumping, lifting, running, and jumping takes a toll on your muscles and joints. You need to stretch them to keep them fluid and to lengthen muscle tissue after all those contractions. Flexible joints and muscles improve range of motion, enabling you to bend and stretch more easily. Stretching helps your balance, decreases your risk of injury, and improves sports performance. (Stretching exercises are coming up later in this chapter.)

every move counts

What's necessary and what's not

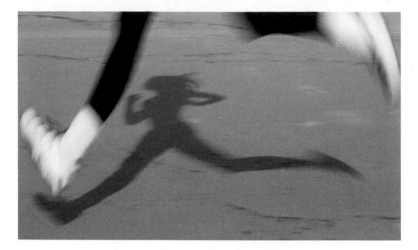

Does the thought of exercise make you ache, gasp for breath, and sweat without even getting off the couch? Relax. You don't have to run a 5-minute mile every day or bench-press 200 pounds to benefit from physical activity. You certainly don't have to be an athlete. You start slow, learn the moves, and build your way up.

Exercise doesn't have to be excruciating—or even strenuous. What *should* it be? That's a function of three things. The first two are pretty straightforward: **Frequency,** how often you do the activity. **Duration,** the length of time you do it. And **intensity,** which refers to how much stress, or overload, is on your body during exercise.

You can measure intensity by counting how fast your heart beats during an activity, how you feel, or by how many calories you burn. What's low intensity for a trained athlete may be high intensity to someone who is just getting started.

While even low intensity activities (like gardening) provide some health benefits, you need moderately intense aerobic activity for 30 to 60 minutes, three to five days a week, for significant health improvement. Better still, vigorous physical activity—working out three to five days a week for 20 to 60 minutes—is the best way to go for cardio fitness. But don't get scared off, *any* increase in your exercise level is a victory!

Strength training is less demanding of your time. Work out your major muscle groups no more than two or three times a week (see the details in Chapter 6). Stretching is flexible. Try to stretch your major muscle groups at least two or three times a week.

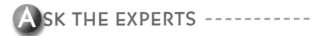

ASK THE EXPERTS

I can barely find 20 minutes free during the day. I can't possibly exercise for 40 minutes straight. What to do?

Not to worry. Your aerobic activity doesn't have to be continuous for you to benefit. You can break it up. The only caveat is that each aerobic session be at least 10 minutes long (plus your warm-up and cool-down). Say you want 30 minutes of aerobics a day. If you can't fit the 30 minutes into one session, split it into two 15-minute sessions. You will, however, get more benefits from one sustained session.

playing it safe

Remember to warm up and cool down

Begin every workout with a five minute warm-up. You want to target the muscles you'll be using in your session. Simply start your exercise but at a much slower pace. For example, use lower gears on your bike, or walk or jog slowly instead of running. Slowly increase your exertion to raise your body temperature and prime your muscles, joints, and circulatory system. The warm-up stage is like warming up your car on a harsh winter day. You shouldn't just start the engine and go. Instead, you should let the engine idle, allowing oil and other necessary fluids to circulate throughout the main systems.

The first month you exercise, keep your workout short and easy. Work up to 50 percent of your maximum heart rate (review *Shaping Up* for a refresher) and try to sustain that for at least 30 minutes. To keep injuries at bay, gradually increase the length of time and the intensity of your workout.

Keep in mind the 10 percent rule: don't hike intensity or duration more than 10 percent a week, and don't hike them both on the same day. Never strength-train the same muscles two days in a row —let yourself recover from the previous day's exertion. Stagger the intensity of your aerobic workouts—hard-to-intense one day, easy-to-moderate the next.

RICE TO THE RESCUE

Suddenly injured? Remember **RICE** which stands for **rest, ice, compression,** and **elevation**. If you suffer a sprain, rest the injured area for a few days. (Don't stop exercising. Just do something that will not aggravate the injury.) Ice the affected area to reduce swelling and pain. (Use an ice pack or a bag of frozen vegetables. Don't put ice cubes on your skin.) Ice for about 20 minutes at least three times a day, for as many days as you feel pain. Compression via an Ace bandage or special wrap sometimes helps keep swelling down, but don't wrap anything until you check with a doctor. Try to keep your injured body part elevated to reduce swelling and help your body carry away waste products around the injury.

If your pain doesn't disappear after a couple of days of RICE, get the injury examined. If you're sidelined for a week or more, decrease your workout by half and work your way back up.

Beating the Heat

You're jogging farther than ever before, mowing the lawn in record time, or chasing tennis balls like you did when you were 14. Be careful—the sun silently zaps your hydration and energy. Soon you might be flat out with heat cramps, heat exhaustion, or heat stroke—which can be fatal. If you feel clumsy or begin to stumble, have a headache, are dizzy, nauseated, sweating excessively or have stopped sweating, by all means stop exercising. Lie down in the shade and drink water. If you start to become confused, or if you have hot, dry skin, seek medical help immediately.

During the summer or in hot climates try to limit workouts to early morning or evening when the sun isn't as hot. Whenever you exercise outdoors, wear sunscreen, a hat appropriate to the season, and sunglasses. Always carry water.

End each workout with a cool-down. Don't stop abruptly, because it can jolt your body unmercifully, triggering dizziness and muscle soreness. Gradually reduce your exertion to help your systems return to normal. Hydrate your body. Dehydration, a decrease in your body's water level, impedes circulation. Two hours before you exercise, drink at least two eight-ounce glasses of water. Drink five ounces more every 15 minutes you exercise. Don't wait until you're thirsty—by then you could already be dehydrated. (Symptoms include weakness, confusion, dry skin that lacks elasticity, an increase in your heart rate and breathing, and a decrease in your blood pressure.)

stretching the benefits

Put some flex time at the end of your workout

When it comes to shaping up, stretching tends to get overlooked. Stretching—simple, painless, quick, and free—erases daily damage to muscles. Imagine your muscles as rubber bands. The ones that have been languishing in the drawer aren't as pliable as the ones used on a regular basis. The unused ones are more apt to snap and tear. Stretched muscles react and contract freely, resulting in a body more supple and natural, free of stiffness and even pain. Stretching increases your range of motion and boosts your strength. And stretching not only improves coordination and workout performance, but also shrinks recovery time between workouts. How? Stretching disperses lactic acid and other waste products that build up in the muscles when you exercise them.

You don't need special clothing, equipment, or even a chunk of time to stretch. In fact, you can do it right now. Put this book down for a moment. Take a slow, deep breath. Exhale and reach for the clouds with a slow, languorous roll of your arms, wrists, and shoulders. Now, stretch your arms out to your sides and turn your palms up, then down. Doesn't that feel good? No wonder. Stretching relieves tension, too, freeing your movement and improving circulation. During a stretch, visualize yourself as trim and fit. Enjoy the process. Done slowly and deliberately, stretching feels great!

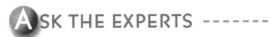

ASK THE EXPERTS

Am I supposed to stretch before or after I work out?

The jury is out on whether or not stretching at the beginning of a workout (after a warm-up, of course) helps prevent injuries. However, it does help alert your muscles to the fact that they're about to go into action. The best time to stretch is at the end of your workout during the cool-down, as it helps elongate the muscles that have just been contracting, and staves off cramps, tightness, and soreness.

Where should I stretch?

You can stretch anywhere, anytime—at your desk, in the car, at the gym. You can easily combine stretching with other activities such as watching TV. You don't need to warm up if all you want to do is a gentle limbering to loosen muscles that stiffen during the course of the day. Just be sure not to force anything, as that invites injury.

stretching head to toe

Doing it right

Regardless of what area of the body you're stretching, ease into it—never bounce. Inhale before you begin, exhale, and relax into the stretch. Hold your stretch for 10 to 15 seconds, less if you're new to stretching or you're uncomfortable. Never force the movement beyond mild resistance. Otherwise, you risk activating the stretch reflex, which makes your muscles contract instead of extend, and defeats the purpose of stretching in the first place. If what you're doing hurts, stop immediately.

Repeat each stretch three to five times. You probably will be able to stretch a tad farther with each repetition. Try to stretch 10 minutes a day, at least three to five days a week, especially after exercise.

Neck

Sit or stand and ease your right ear toward your right shoulder. Gently lower the left shoulder. With the fingers of your right hand, gently nudge your head closer to your right shoulder. Release, then do the other side. When you're done, shrug your shoulders, hold, and release.

Face forward. Slowly turn your head right, stopping at the point of resistance. Hold. Gradually return to the middle, then repeat left, and return to the middle. After you finish, drop your chin to your chest (keeping your shoulders back), hold, and release.

Shoulders

Stand or sit and extend your right arm straight across your chest. Take your left hand and hug your right elbow into your chest. Hold, release, then switch arms and repeat.

Stand or sit and raise one arm straight up over your head and stretch it as far as you can without bending your body. Open your palm upwards and push toward the ceiling a couple of times, then

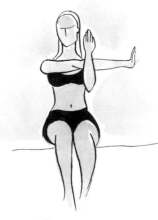

release and repeat with the other arm. To include your torso in the stretch, as you reach with your right arm, bend to the left at your waist. Hold, release, then switch sides and repeat.

Triceps

Stand or sit and reach your right arm up and behind your head as if to scratch your back. (Your arm will form an inverted V by your ear.) With your left hand, reach over your head and slowly pull down the elbow of your right arm. Hold, release, switch arms and repeat.

Biceps

Extend your right arm out in front of you, palm up. With your left hand, grasp the fingers of your right hand and tug them toward the floor, keep your right arm straight in front of you, parallel to the floor. Switch arms and repeat.

Forearms

Stand or sit and extend your right arm out in front of you, palm facing down. With your other hand, grab the fingers of your right hand and gently tug them toward your shoulder. Hold, release, switch arms and repeat.

Chest

Stand tall and clasp your hands behind your back. Squeeze your shoulder blades toward each other and lift your chest up and out, raising your hands and arms a bit if you can. Try not to arch your lower back. Hold, release, and repeat.

Stand in a doorway with your right arm bent in a 90-degree angle at the elbow, your right forearm resting against the doorframe. Slowly lean forward until you feel a comfortable stretch in your chest muscles. Hold, release, and repeat on the other side.

stretching *(cont'd.)*

Back

Lie on your back, legs extended. Slowly bend your right knee, clasp it with your hands, and pull it toward your chest (as far as you can without discomfort). Hold. Slowly release. Switch legs and repeat. When you're done, hug both knees to your chest, hold, and release.

Get on your hands and knees, eyes looking forward. Exhale slowly and let your head slowly sag toward the floor while you arch your back toward the ceiling. Hold in your stomach muscles ("abs"). Hold, then release, allowing your back to sag.

To stretch your upper back, sit or stand and extend your arms in front of you at shoulder height, your fingers clasped together. Drop your head, turn your palms out, round your shoulders and back, and reach your arms out even farther. Hold and release.
To stretch the muscles that run alongside your back, stand up (feet shoulder-width apart), interlace your fingers, turn your palms up, and reach toward the ceiling. Slowly bend to one side. Hold, then return to the middle. Repeat on the other side.

Calves

Stand up, extend your arms in front of you, and put your hands shoulder-width apart on a wall. Step back a couple of feet. Keep your legs straight, feet and heels on the floor, and lean into the wall. Hold and release. (For a variation, put one leg forward, slightly bent, and the other behind you, as straight as possible, then lean.)

Holding onto a railing or the back of a chair, stand on a step and allow your heels to hang off the edge, lower than your toes. Slowly raise up on your toes for several seconds, then slowly lower your weight onto your heels. To spice things up a little, shift your weight from one heel to the next. These calf stretches help prevent shin splints, too.

Ankles

Sit on a chair and extend your legs out in front of you, your feet one or two inches off the ground. Flex your ankles and feet toward you and hold, then slowly point your toes and feet away from you and downward, and hold.

EASE INTO IT

Tonight, instead of plopping onto the couch when it's time for your favorite TV show, hike around the room and swing your arms while those first few commercials are on. Then when the show starts, ease onto the floor, kick off your shoes and socks, and do the stretching exercises on pages 116-119. You'll be done and feeling great before the end credits roll!

equipping your home gym

Home sweat home

You don't need a turbo-charged treadmill to stay in shape at home, but exercise equipment sure can make your workout more convenient and interesting. What types of equipment should you get? Whatever complements your workout program. For example, if you love to run outside, you probably don't need fancy cardio equipment. Your money might be better spent on free weights or a multi-gym (see *Chapter 6* for everything you need to know about strength-training equipment), a few exercise tapes, and a jump rope. If you hate to exercise outdoors and the gym isn't for you, aim for something that works your cardio fitness, like a treadmill, bike, rower, stairclimber, or ski machine.

While they'll all work your heart, machines can be as different as a VW Bug and a Lexus. Before you buy anything, drag yourself to the gym on a day pass and work out on the equipment. Many machines offer preset programs that automatically vary speed, resistance, distance, and time. With others you can program your own workouts. Note the machines and features you like, be realistic about which you will most likely use, then do some research. Go to the library or online (www.ask.com is a good place to start), and search for the latest reviews on the specific type of machine that interests you.

Next, head to the fitness stores. You'll need to run another check, as residential fitness equipment tends to have a much different feel than commercial machines.

Bells and whistles such as calorie-counters and heart monitors are fun, but they tend to be expensive and inaccurate when built into machines. If you can't manage to take your pulse while exercising, buy a separate heart monitor.

Before you buy, call the customer support number to see if someone will actually explain things to you. If no one does, cross that brand off the list. Make sure whatever you buy comes with a warranty and that you'll be able to have the machine serviced conveniently. Ask for a total price that includes tax, delivery, shipping, and set-up. It can't hurt to check the classifieds to see if there's a gently used model of what you're looking for. (Try it out first—carefully—as you don't know what kind of shape it's really in.) The bottom line: never buy an exercise machine you haven't tried out first.

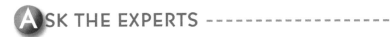

ASK THE EXPERTS

Where's the best place to put exercise equipment?

Somewhere you can safely and comfortably work out where you won't be disturbed by (or disturb) your mate, your roommate, or your kids. (Make sure your little ones can't turn on the equipment by themselves.) You'll need space with adequate head room, ventilation, lighting, and proximity to the TV or the stereo (to make your workout more pleasant.) A mirror will help you assess your technique. Consider putting a mat under the equipment to reduce noise and wear and tear on the floor.

With so many exercise tapes out there, how do I know which ones will work for me?

Before you buy a videotape, check it out. You can borrow tapes from a friend or your library, or rent them from the video store. You can find reviews online at www.exercisevideosreviews.com and www.collagevideo.com.

wearing the right gear

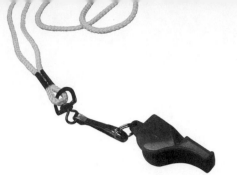

Don't let your clothes leave you hanging

You don't need to spend lots of money on clothes and footwear in order to exercise. But you do need to make sure the clothing fits the workout. Before you grab your garb, address these issues:

Mobility. Will the clothes allow you the freedom to move during your workout or will they restrict you? Make sure whatever you wear won't get caught in the equipment being used.

Comfort. Will you be too hot or too cold? If it's cold outside, wear gloves or mittens, a hat that covers your ears, and something to warm your face. Whether you're indoors or out, wear layers that you can peel off as you warm up. If you're a woman, wear an exercise bra for extra support.

Self-consciousness. If you don't feel comfortable doing the thong thing, why do it? You can get the same workout wearing a T-shirt with your favorite pizzeria's logo on it. (Hey, maybe the T-shirt will even motivate you. "If I spend five more minutes on this treadmill every day, I'm going to have pizza with my salad on Friday night!") If you want to show off your efforts in a thong, go for it!

Safety. If you exercise outside at night or in fog, will you be seen? Make sure to wear brightly colored clothing, preferably with reflective stripes. If you're exercising in the street, can you hear? Much as it's oh-so-invigorating to hoof it accompanied by Ricky Martin on your headphones, just check to make sure you can hear oncoming cars. Carry a police whistle in your pocket, in case you're in danger or get hurt and can't yell for help. It doesn't hurt to carry a cell phone either.

EXERCISE ON THE RIGHT FOOT

If you can buy only one piece of gear, make it a pair of good shoes. When you work out, you need something that can stand up to a pounding. The wrong shoe can hinder performance and endanger your safety. Flimsy sneakers, for example, don't give the proper arch support crucial to a safe workout. Running shoes are treacherous in step or aerobics class. They don't provide adequate support during lateral movements, and leave you open to falls and sprains. To get the right shoes, figure out what exercise you'll be doing most. If you plan to do the same activity twice or more a week, get a specific shoe for that activity. If you plan on something different each day or can afford only one type of shoe, get a cross-trainer.

Go to an athletic-shoe store, and ask a salesperson to help find a shoe that fits your needs. If you have high arches, for example, you'll need good shock absorbers. If you have low arches, you'll need more support in the heel. If you over-pronate (your foot rolls inward too much) or supinate (your foot rolls outward), look for motion-control shoes or get fitted for orthotics with good shock absorption in the arch.

Try on shoes at the end of the day, when your foot size is largest, and wear your workout socks. Try on both shoes, as one foot might be bigger than the other. (Buy the bigger size.) Hike around in the store. Shoes should be comfortable from the outset. (Your toes should be able to wiggle in them.) If the shoes don't feel great, don't get them.

picking a gym

Do you belong with the thonged throngs?

You're about to pop a step video into the VCR when suddenly the phone is ringing, the kids need help with their homework, the cat is choking on a Lego. Sometimes, in spite of best intentions, exercising at home seems impossible. That's when you realize the gym may be a better option.

There's also a great collection of equipment, classes, and professional guidance at the gym, fostering a workout that's varied, challenging, and interesting. There's the chance to socialize with others, which you don't get at home in front of your "Biceps of Iron" videotape. If you work out during lunch hour or on either end of your workday, the gym might be much more convenient. And your employer might pick up part of the gym tab.

Health clubs tend to have unique personalities that may or may not fit yours. To narrow the prospects, first figure out when you're most likely to exercise. Then draw up a list of gyms by location—closer to home or work depending on when you plan to work out. There's no sense picking a gym across town from work, for example, if you hope to squeeze a workout into the lunch hour.

Then go exploring to see if you feel comfortable. Most gyms let you sign up for a day or two for free or for a nominal fee. Look for free weights, weight machines, and cardiovascular equipment. Make

FIRST-PERSON DISASTER

I visited a local health club on the weekend and thought I'd found Nirvana: no lines, lots of classes and equipment, even nutrition counseling. I signed up for a one-year membership. When Monday came around, I dropped my daughter off at school and headed for the gym. I had to circle the parking lot four times before I found a space. When I finally got to the kickboxing class I signed up for when I joined, it was so jammed, I kept smacking my arm into the guy next to me. It was not a pleasant experience. I wish I'd visited during the time I planned to exercise!

Doug J., Hoboken, New Jersey

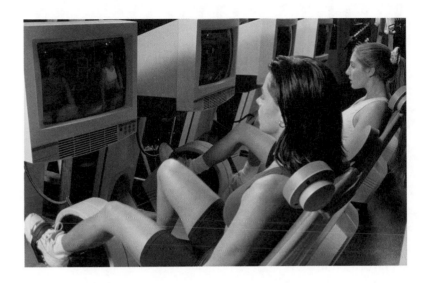

sure everything's in working order. Community centers such as the YMCA often offer basketball and racquetball courts and a pool, but may lack state-of-the-art equipment and classes available at more expensive clubs. If you're bent on yoga, kickboxing, and spinning and all a gym offers is step class, find another gym. Talk to other members whose fitness levels seem to match yours, and watch how the staff interacts with the clientele. The staff should be certified by accredited fitness groups and should be there to serve all, not just to cozy up to the buff bods.

Check out the locker room. Would you want to take a shower there? Does it have a suitable place to hang your Donna Karan suit while you sweat? Is everything clean and in working order? List amenities such as babysitting, parking, laundry service, lockers, hair dryers, massage, personal training, and nutrition help, which can make life easier. When the gym takes care of the whole you, you're less likely to drop out.

finding a personal trainer

Take your cue from Madonna and Brad Pitt

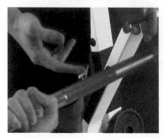

Whether you work out at home or in the gym, consider enlisting a little help from a fitness pro to get you moving in the right direction. A personal trainer will assess your fitness before you even break a sweat. Then she'll custom-design workouts to help meet your goals. She'll guide you through the moves correctly and safely, help choose equipment, keep track of workouts, and make sure you progress at your own pace. She'll even design a program around your favorite music.

All this convenience comes with a price—from $30 to $100 an hour. The price tag might seem steep until you consider that it's an investment in your fitness future. It's also a great motivator. When the trainer shows up at the door, you know she's not carrying crullers and coffee in that gym bag. There's no sense ducking behind the couch and closing the blinds—if you cancel in less than 24 hours before the session, you usually have to pay anyway. So you drag yourself off the couch, and before you know it, you're moving and energized.

FITNESS FACTS

About Those Miracle Machines on TV...

All you have to do is channel-surf for a couple of minutes and you see them—those hard bodies whose abs could substitute for the washboard in a country music band. "All you have to do is use Miracle Muscles for three minutes a day and you, too, can look like this . . ." The announcer fails to mention everything else you'd have to do to look like that. No machine or exercise can burn fat off a particular part of your body. Nothing gets you into shape in only three minutes a day. To get real results, you have to eat smart and put work into the workout.

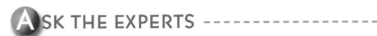

ASK THE EXPERTS

Don't get me wrong—I would love to have a personal trainer help me work out, but there's no way I can afford it. Are there ways around this problem?

Yes. If you can't afford regular sessions, hire the trainer for a few sessions to design a program and walk you through the proper steps of the routine. Or work with the trainer every other week for a few months and make sure to do your homework between visits. You also can split the cost with a friend or two and have sessions together. For example, you and a couple of other at-home moms and dads in the neighborhood can get together and have the trainer visit each week. Alternatively, you and your colleagues or gym pals can meet with the trainer at the health club and split the fee.

My dog groomer is suddenly calling herself a personal trainer. How do I know who's reputable and who's not?

Check the pro's credentials. A reputable gym, university, or hospital should be able to hook you up with an instructor certified by a legitimate fitness group. Check for someone with a degree in physical education or certified from a group such as the American College of Sports Medicine, the National Strength and Conditioning Association, the IDEA Foundation, the Association of Fitness Professionals, the Aerobic Fitness Association of America, the National Academy of Sports Medicine, the American Council on Exercise, the National Dance Exercise Instructors Training Association, the National Academy of Sports Medicine, or the Institute for Aerobics Research.

now what do I do?

Answers to common questions

Q I've signed up for exercise classes in the past, only to quit after one or two because I felt like a klutz. Why can't I get it?

Unless you're a prima donna or a preschooler, it's not every day you twirl and kick and jump, often at the same time. Give yourself a couple of weeks to get used to the moves. At the same time, don't be afraid to ask for help. Outside class, ask the instructor to break down the moves for you, or watch a similar class that she teaches. If you get stuck during class, or you feel too winded to keep up, eliminate the arm movements and jog in place until you get back into sync.

Sign up for a class that not only suits your fitness level, but also one that addresses your familiarity with the techniques. Once you master the techniques you can build up the intensity. Just as you wouldn't step into a ring with Mike Tyson without preparation (even with it!), you can't expect to jump into an intense, high-energy workout like cardio kickboxing, spend 45 minutes kicking and punching with ballistic speed, and go home standing. The movements are unfamiliar, they require a certain amount of conditioning, and if you do them wrong, you're apt to pull or even tear your muscles.

In a class or in the gym, don't let machismo overpower common sense. You might be tempted to enroll in advanced spinning class, even though you're a novice, because, hey, you're a CEO with stock options and there's nothing you can't do. But if you haven't worked up to that level, you risk doing damage.

Q Will I lose weight just by increasing my physical activity?

Yes, even if you don't reduce your caloric intake, you can lose weight by stepping up your activity. (Of course, you can't increase your calorie intake at the same time and expect to lose.) If you increase your physical activity and decrease your caloric intake, you'll lose weight more quickly. Being physically active will help you maintain your weight loss as well.

BOOKS

ACSM Fitness Book, Steven Blair
A beginner's guide to a sound exercise program. Easy-to-use, color-coded system takes you through a variety of routines.

Fitness for Dummies, Liz Neporent and Suzanne Schlosberg
A thorough, entertaining guide to fitness, including tips, techniques, and strategies for testing your fitness level, setting your goals, designing routines that meet your needs, and sticking with your program.

EQUIPMENT

www.ask.com
In the question box, just type in the kind of fitness equipment you're looking for and then navigate to reviews and price guides.

www.bodytrends.com
Treadmills, elliptical trainers, heart-rate monitors, free weights, videos, and information on how to choose and use the equipment.

VIDEOS

Karen Voight's Pure & Simple Stretch
Beginner-intermediate stretch. Increase your flexibility accompanied by flute and guitar music.

Gay Gasper's NutraBody Workout
Beginner-intermediate, low impact. Includes a.m. aerobics and p.m. toning for men and women. Requires dumbbells and exercise tube.

Millennium Stretch with Scott Cole
Intermediate stretching routine incorporates yoga, tai chi, and other Eastern mind/body techniques with Western stretches. Very soothing and relaxing.

WEB SITES

www.acefitness.com
Site of American Council on Exercise, a non-profit group committed to promoting active lifestyles and physical fitness. For information or referral by phone, call 800-825-3636.

www.acsm.org
Site of the American College of Sports Medicine, which offers resources on fitness, including free brochures on topics ranging from eating smart to fitness over age 40. Contact them at 317-637-9200.

www.healthclubs.com
Offers advice on how to choose a health club. Finds health clubs in or near your town that cater to specific needs.

6

pumping up

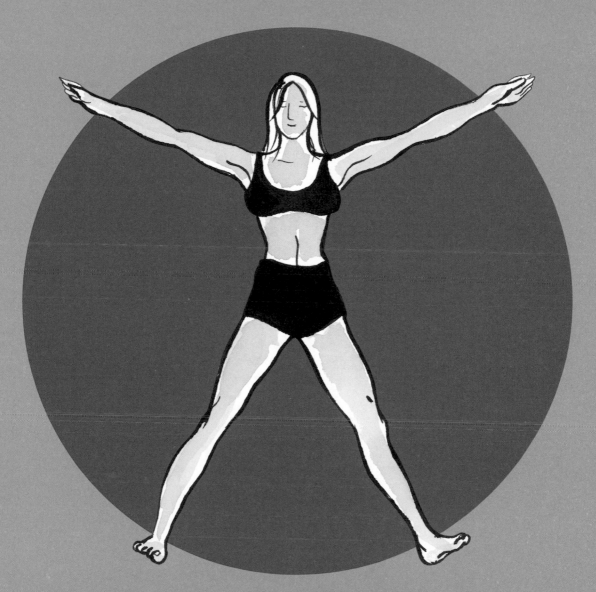

Just about anybody can do strength training—
in less time than it takes to watch the evening
news. And after only a month or so of working
with weights, you'll like the results so much,
you'll wonder why you waited so long to try it!

get pumped

Lifting weights produces almost immediate results

Lifting weights is one of the most popular fitness activities in America. But you don't need to be a bodybuilder to reap the benefits. What does strength training have to offer? Plenty!

Strength training (a.k.a. **weight** or **resistance training**) is an essential part of getting in shape. It strengthens and tones your muscles, making them firmer and denser while improving muscular endurance. Without strength training, you lose muscle mass as you age.

As you grow older, bone density decreases, hiking your risk of **osteoporosis**, a bone disorder that increases the risk of fractures. Studies show that weight training slows bone loss and even increases bone density. This is particularly important for women, who experience bone loss of about .7 to 1.0 percent a year after age 30.

FITNESS FACTS

Endurance vs. Strength

Muscular strength is a muscle's ability to generate force. It's what you need for things like lugging that giant stack of books over to your tag sale pile. **Muscular endurance** is the ability of a muscle to generate force repeatedly. That's important in sports like tennis and for activities such as waxing your car and lifting your baby in and out—and in and out—of his car seat. Generally speaking, training for muscular strength will also increase muscle endurance. But training for muscular endurance doesn't significantly increase muscular strength.

MORE STRENGTHS OF STRENGTH TRAINING

Strength training improves your:
- Flexibility and mobility
- Glucose metabolism (a factor in managing and preventing some forms of diabetes)
- Performance in sports and other physical activities
- Posture
- Self-esteem and mood
- Personal appearance

It also:
- Helps control blood pressure
- Reduces the incidence of lower-back pain
- Decreases arthritic pain
- Reduces joint and muscle injuries
- Makes everyday tasks easier

Strength training also thickens and strengthens tendons, ligaments, and other connective tissue around muscles. It helps you maintain and lose weight. When you strength train, you work your muscles against resistance in the form of free weights, machines, elastic tubes or bands, or your own weight—pushing your muscles beyond what they do in an average day. As a result, you develop more muscle mass, which requires more energy (calories) to support than fat does. Muscle burns 17 to 25 times as many calories as fat, so the more muscle you develop, the more calories you burn— even when you're sleeping!

Strength training for as little as 20 minutes, two days a week gives you all this and more (read on)—without breaking the bank!

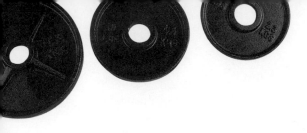

getting started

*What pumps
you up?*

So you want to start a strength-training program. Great. But first, ask yourself what's motivating you? Is it health concerns? Do you want to look great in that new shirt? Improve your tennis game? Figure out your motivation and keep reminding yourself of it, since that's the essence of sticking with any program.

If you're new to strength training, you have an advantage over someone who's been at it for a while. Within a few weeks of starting your program, you'll see exciting changes in your body—and in your strength. Someone who's already muscularly fit won't see such dramatic progress during the same period.

Even so, no matter how motivated you are, you're less apt to stick with strength training if you're not having fun—and if it's not convenient. You're in luck. All you need is 20 minutes, two or three times a week, to get your muscles in shape. Fit this into your lunch hour or while you're watching TV.

Figure out how to make strength training fun. For some people, it's working out with a partner. (A partner can also spot you, check your form, and spur you on.) Others prefer to exercise alone. For some, cranking up Santana does the trick; for others, it's peace and quiet that gets them moving.

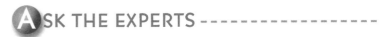

ASK THE EXPERTS

I'm a woman. Will I end up looking like the Incredible Hulk if I strength-train?

No, women can't develop muscles like men. Women don't have nearly the amount of testosterone (the male sex hormone that builds muscles) that men have. If you strength-train, your muscles will look toned, not bulky.

Which should I do first: aerobics or strength training?

You can do them in either order. But if you're focusing on strength training, do that first so your muscles aren't tired out from the aerobic workout. Conversely, if aerobics is what you're concentrating on, do that first.

OVERCOMING RESISTANCE

How Many Muscles Do You Have?

Don't know the answer? You have more than 600 muscles. Most of them are skeletal muscles, which provide force to move your body and maintain posture—the ones you'll work out by strength training. They're actually a collection of fibers that respond to nerve messages by contracting and pulling on your bones—which makes you move.

A muscle won't get stronger or bigger unless resistance is applied to it and the muscle is forced to work harder. That's what strength training does. It works your muscles against force or outside resistance, such as weights. (That's why it's also called resistance training.) Your muscles have to overcome resistance against gravity and do their job.

equipping yourself

Free weights and machines

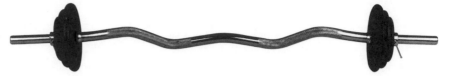

Chances are, you'll want to start strength-training with free weights. Free weights are bars with weights on both ends. There are two kinds: **dumbbells** and **barbells.** Dumbbells, short bars with weights on the ends, weigh one to 180 pounds and are a good choice for beginners. Some are one-piece and others are adjustable, which means the weights attach by collars, pins, magnets, or screws so you can vary the load. Barbells are six- to seven-foot bars that weigh anywhere from 15 to 45 pounds. One or more weights—called **plates**—slide onto the bars. Plates, which are secured by **collars,** range from one to 45 pounds.

A good way for women to start is with dumbbells weighing 2, 3, 5, 8, 10, 12, and 15 pounds. For men: use 8-, 12-, 15-, 20-, 25-, 30-, 35-, and 40-pound weights. Dumbbells or plates with multi-sided edges are a good choice.

Machines are another way to go. For home use, the most versatile machines are **multi-gyms,** which have multiple stations that allow you to perform a variety of exercises. Some multi-gyms cost $400 or so, but better-quality units start around $1,000. Multi-gyms usually have one or two weight stacks; the second stack allows another person to use the gym at the same time. One-stack machines typically require about 15 feet of floor space; two-stack machines need more than twice that.

Look for gyms with stations such as knee raises, chest and shoulder presses, leg presses, leg extensions, and curls. Consider gyms that let you switch stations without having to hook and unhook cables. And try a machine before you buy it: make sure it fits your body, that cables and pulleys operate smoothly and quietly, and that the seat is sturdy and adequately padded. (See *Fitness that fits* for tips on buying exercise machines.)

Free Weights vs. Machines

Ah, the great debate. Some experts recommend starting out with machines because they keep your body in the correct position and guide it through the correct motions. Machines better isolate specific muscles, making your workout more effective. They're generally safer than free weights, which can fall on you. Finally, machines don't require as much coordination and balance as free weights do.

Free weights, on the other hand, are less expensive and take up less room than most machines. Unlike machines, free weights can be used by people of any size. Free weights allow you to do hundreds of exercises and work out more dimensions of your muscles. And because they often work several muscle groups at the same time, free-weight exercises more closely simulate the way your muscles work in real life. It's easier to use poor form with free weights, though, and harder to get the hang of them. You should use a spotter if you're new to free weights, especially if they're heavy.

You might want to consider working out with machines and free weights—for the benefits of each and for variety. Whatever equipment you use, remember that it's not the type of equipment that determines how much you get from strength training, but how you use it.

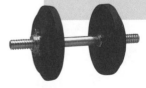

gearing up

Accessorize your workout

If you're using free weights, a bench is a great investment. Your body will appreciate the padding and you'll get more out of some of the exercises. A bench allows you to move through the full range of motion (the entire arc that a muscle can move through). You'll be able to lower your elbow below body level for certain exercises, which you can't do if you're on the floor. You can buy a flat, upright, or adjustable bench, depending on what exercises you'll be doing and how much you want to spend. They range from about $50 to $600. Before purchasing a bench, be sure it's stable, wide enough for your body, and allows your feet to touch the floor when lying on your back.

For nice and tidy storage of dumbbells, consider buying a **rack**. They start at around $100. For your barbells, buy either a rack (starting at $75) or a weight tree (from $75 up).

Be kind to your body and buy an **exercise mat** for floor exercises—especially if your floor has no padding. Look for one that's washable and folds up. Mats start around $20.

Some lower-body exercises call for **ankle weights** ($15 to $40). You can buy a range of weights or an adjustable pair.

Strength-training gloves are a good idea if you're lifting heavy weights. They protect hands from calluses, cushion palms, and help keep your grip if your hands are sweaty. Some feature a wrap for wrist support and stability. Gloves start at $10.

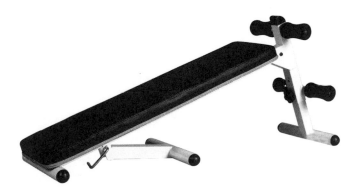

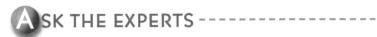
Where can I buy strength-training equipment?

Try a sporting goods store or a store specializing in fitness equipment. Medical supply stores often carry exercise bands. Check out the Internet. (See the resources at the end of this chapter.)

Should I use dumbbells or barbells?

If you're a beginner, start with dumbbells. If you lift heavy weights, go with barbells. Keep in mind that you need two hands to lift a barbell, which means you may end up relying on your stronger side to lift it. With dumbbells, you generally use only one hand at a time, which gives you a more balanced workout.

FITNESS FACTS

Elastic Resistance

Elastic exercise bands and tubing offer portable, inexpensive ($3 to $20) resistance. Bands are elastic straps; tubing is elastic cording, often with handles on each end. Elastic resistance challenges your muscles in a different way. Because bands and tubes will snap back at you if you don't stay in control (ouch!), they force you to focus on the lifting and lowering parts of an exercise. But they won't build as much strength as machines and free weights. Some companies sell bands and tubes in sets with varying amounts of tension (resistance). Consider buying door attachments and ankle straps for tubing. Be sure to check for holes and splits that can develop over time. These are great for on-the-road maintenance.

reps, sets, and resistance

How much to do

Weight trainers are always throwing around words like "reps" and "sets." A **rep**, or repetition, is one (complete) sequence of an exercise. For example, one rep of a side raise is lifting weights out to your sides and lowering them once. A **set** is a series of reps done without resting. A set of side raises, for example, might be 10 reps.

How many reps and sets should you do? Keep in mind that the only way to increase muscle strength and endurance is to challenge muscles to work harder than they're used to. It's what exercise gurus call the overload principle. However, many experts say that if you're strength-training for fitness—moderate increases in muscle mass, strength, and endurance—one set of 10 to 12 reps for each of the major muscle groups is sufficient.

If you want to continue to gain muscle strength and size, you'll need to do more sets (two or three), use heavier weights, and decrease your reps. You should struggle to complete 12 reps or the workout is not heavy enough.

If muscle endurance (as opposed to strength) is what you're looking for—you have your eye on winning the local tennis championship,

FIRST-PERSON DISASTER

I used to lift weights five times a week. One day at the gym, I was bench-pressing 200 pounds. As I lifted the barbell, I felt something snap on the right side of my chest. It was as if someone had kicked me. My right arm dropped, the plates fell off one side of the bar—I didn't have collars on—and the bar flew across the gym.

Luckily, no one else was hurt. I ended up with a ruptured tendon in my pectoral muscle. After six months of therapy, I returned to weight training. Now I strength train three days a week and give my muscles a day off between workouts. I learned about overtraining the hard way!

—Michael T., Pasadena, California

for instance—experts recommend increasing your reps (to 15 or more), decreasing the resistance (weight), and doing multiple sets. How much weight should you use? The right amount of weight, or resistance, is one that makes your muscles feel exhausted by the end of each set. This is known as working muscles "to fatigue."

Start with a weight, say, three pounds. If you feel you can keep going—with good form and technique—after 12 reps, it's too light. If you can't make it to 10 reps, it's too heavy. The right weight is one you can lift 12 times but challenges you to keep good form and technique for the last one or two reps. It may take a few sessions before you find the one that fits the bill.

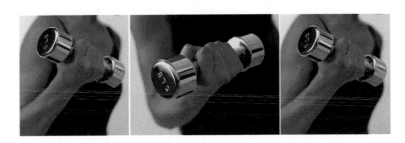

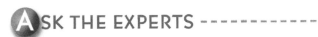

ASK THE EXPERTS

Which muscles should I work out?

Your training sessions should exercise the major muscle groups: the front and back of your arms, your chest, shoulders, abdomen, back and buttocks, the front and back of your thighs, and your calves.

doing it right

*Tips for
a successful,
and safe,
program*

The key to successful strength training isn't how many pounds you lift. It's how you lift them. Here's how to do it right:

- Warm up with five to 10 minutes of aerobic exercise involving your arms and legs (like brisk walking). Lightly stretch the muscles you'll use. Stretch for five to 10 minutes after each session to maintain flexibility, avoid soreness, and reduce the risk of injury. (See the stretches in *Fitness that fits*.)
- Perform reps slowly. Rushing increases your risk of injury and makes your workout less efficient. Feel the entire move. Take two seconds to lift a weight (count "one, 1,000, two, 1,000") and four seconds to lower it.

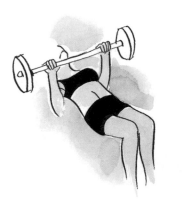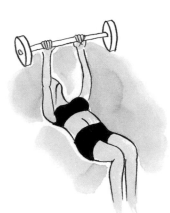

- Pause between lifting and lowering. Focus on the muscle.
- Do each rep in a controlled and deliberate way. This lessens the risk of injury and makes sure muscle, not momentum, is doing the work. When lowering a weight, don't let gravity accelerate it.
- Breathe! Exhale when you exert effort; inhale when you lower or release, keeping your breathing even and smooth. Never hold your breath—it can raise your blood pressure.
- Flex the muscle you're working; relax the others. Don't clench your fists or tighten your face.
- Don't skip the difficult parts of an exercise.
- Maintain a slight bend in your elbows and knees. Don't bend your back.

- To maintain balance, keep your eyes open. Watch yourself in a mirror or focus on something in the distance.
- Use a spotter when using heavy free weights.
- Wait one to three minutes between sets to give muscles time to recover.
- If you feel pain, stop!
- If your heart rate is more than 100 beats per minute after your session, cool down—walk or slowly pedal a stationary bike, for instance—until your heart rate slows.
- Practice a new exercise with a light weight.
- Wait at least 48 hours between sessions to give muscles time to rebuild. Strength-train the same muscles no more than three times a week. Muscles strengthen between (not during) workouts.
- Get enough sleep to help muscles rebuild.

SEE A PRO

It's a good idea to hire a fitness professional for a few sessions to show you proper weight-training technique and form. A professional also can help design a routine and advise you on purchasing equipment. The *Fitness That Fits* chapter gives you tips on finding a pro.

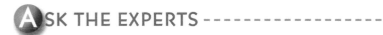ASK THE EXPERTS

Should I keep weight training if I hurt somewhere?

Discomfort or a mild burning sensation in the muscles you work during your routine is normal. It means your body is doing more than it's used to. Expect to feel slightly sore a day or two after your workout—a sign that your muscles are adapting. Pain, on the other hand, means something is wrong. Check your technique. If you still have pain, stop your session. If you have joint pain after your routine, decrease your reps or resistance until you're pain-free for at least two weeks. If the pain persists, call your doctor.

Note: If you've had a previous injury or any conditions noted in *Shaping Up*, seek medical advice before starting a program.

chest and shoulders

*Perk up
your pecs
and develop
your delts*

Now that you know the ins and outs of strength training, get pumped to learn some moves for your major muscle groups. Remember, stop if you feel pain.

Your chest muscles are called **pectorals** or **pecs** (use terms like this to impress everyone!). They cooperate with shoulder muscles to lift your arms and move them forward. You use pecs for just about everything you do with your arms.

Dumbbell Chest Presses (for pecs, deltoids, triceps)
Position: Lie on a bench (less ideally, the floor), facing up, with feet flat on the floor or on the bench. Hold a dumbbell on either side of your chest with your palms facing forward and elbows extended slightly below your shoulders (but not lower than the bench).
Movement: Slowly push up the weights. Your arms should be directly over your shoulders. Hold, then slowly lower.
Tips: Pull in your abdominal muscles. Don't lock your elbows or let your shoulder blades rise off the bench.

Push-ups (for pecs, triceps, deltoids)
Position: Kneel on the floor, face down. Place your hands flat on the floor, fingers facing forward, slightly more than shoulder-width apart. Extend your legs directly behind you, balancing on your toes.
Movement: Slowly push up by straightening your arms. Slowly lower your body until your chest is one to two inches off the ground.
Tips: Keep your abdominals pulled in and maintain one strong line from neck to feet, back straight. Lower your body as a unit. Don't lock your elbows. Exhale on the way up, and inhale as you come down. (If you're not strong enough to do these properly, do standing push-ups by leaning into a wall and pushing forward.)
Alternative: A modified push-up is easier. Bend your legs and balance on your hands and knees (with a mat), keeping your feet off the floor.

Shoulder muscles are called **deltoids** or **delts**. They work with other muscles to lift your arms, move them sideways, and extend them backward. You need delts to lift your little bundle of joy and to throw a baseball. The **rotator cuff** is the group of muscles that keep your arm in its socket. You use them when you throw and catch, and when you raise your arm over your head.

Side Raises (for deltoids, especially the sides)

Position: Stand, or sit on a chair or a bench, with a dumbbell in each hand, arms by your sides and palms facing in.

Movement: Slowly lift your arms straight out to the sides until they're parallel to the floor. Squeeze your delts. Slowly lower.

Tips: Keep your wrists straight and neck relaxed. Don't hunch your shoulders. If you're standing, slightly bend your knees. Don't let the dumbbells extend beyond your shoulders.

Shoulder Presses (for side and rear shoulders, trapezoids)

Position: Sit on a chair or a bench (if adjustable, raise it to 90 degrees), feet flat on the floor (hip-width apart). Hold a dumbbell in each hand next to your shoulders with elbows and palms facing forward. Forearms should be perpendicular to the floor.

Movement: Slowly lift the weights above your head by straightening your arms. Tighten your shoulder muscles. Slowly lower your arms to shoulder level.

Tips: Do the exercise one arm at a time or while standing.

FLEXING YOUR MUSCLE

Most exercises require that you flex (contract, tighten) a particular muscle. To flex, give the muscle a deliberate squeeze. Picture someone coming at you, about to punch you in that muscle—that should make you flex!

arms and upper back

Strong arm tactics

The muscles in the front of your upper arms, the biceps (or **bis**), bend your arm. They help you pick up and carry things. The **triceps** (or **tris**), at the back of your upper arm, help extend your shoulders. Whenever you push something, you use triceps.

Bicep Curls (for bis)

Position: Stand, feet slightly wider than shoulder-width apart, arms by your sides, a weight in each hand, and palms forward.
Movement: Bending your elbows, slowly curl the weights toward your shoulders. Squeeze your biceps as you lift. Slowly lower.
Tips: Keep your shoulders back, wrists strong, elbows close to your sides (not locked), and knees slightly bent. Pull in your abdominal muscles. You can do the curl one arm at a time.

Kickbacks (for tris)

Position: Sitting on a flat bench or a chair, bend at the waist (with a straight back and torso parallel with the floor) with one foot slightly in front of the other. Place a dumbbell in your right hand next to your side, palm facing the side of your thigh. Bend your elbow to form a 90-degree angle with your upper arm parallel with the floor. Place your left hand in front of you on the bench or the chair, elbow extended.
Movement: Slowly extend your right arm fully back (without locking your elbow), raising your forearm. Keep your right elbow close to your side. Flex your triceps. Slowly lower your arm. After completing a set, repeat with the left arm.
Tips: Slightly bend the knee on the side holding the weight. Keep your head in line with your back. Pull in your abdominals.

The **latissimus dorsi** (or **lats**), and the **trapezius** (or **traps**) are two major muscles of the upper back. The lats help pull the shoulders back and downward, and assist in pressing. The traps help you shrug your shoulders and squeeze them together. Your **rhomboids** work with the traps when you squeeze your shoulders together and help you maintain good posture.

Bent Dumbbell Row (upper back muscles, including the rhomboids, also the biceps)

Position: Stand with your right foot 12 inches in front of your left. Lean on a flat bench or a chair with your left arm fully extended. Hold a dumbbell in your right hand and fully extend your arm at your side, palm toward your body. Bend at the waist until your upper body is almost parallel with the floor.

Movement: Slowly pull up your right elbow as high as you can, using your upper back and not your arm muscles. Flex your right upper-back muscles. Slowly return to your starting position. After completing a set, repeat with the left arm.

Tips: Keep your back stable and your neck long, and tighten your abdominals. Movement should skim the side of your body (arms stay close to the body). Don't let the weight drop down. Don't shrug your shoulders.

Upright Rows (for traps and delts)

Position: Stand with your feet a few inches apart, a dumbbell in each hand in front of your upper thighs, palms facing your body.

Movement: Slowly extend your elbows outward, keeping the dumbbell close to your body, and raise to chin height. Squeeze your traps and slowly return to the starting position.

abs and lower back

Abs-olutely marvelous tummy-tuckers

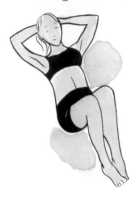

The abdominal muscle group, or abs, consists of four muscles: rectus abdominis, transverse abdominis, and internal and external obliques. The rectus abdominis, the longest abdominal muscle, pulls your upper body toward your lower body. The transverse abdominis contracts when you sneeze or cough. The obliques help you bend side to side, rotate your torso, and bend your body forward. Strong abs not only make you look great, but they help you stand erect, keep your internal organs in place, and prevent lower back pain.

Basic Crunches (for rectus abdominus)

Position: Lie on the floor (face toward the ceiling) with hands one on top of the other behind your head. Don't lace your fingers together; keep elbows out and rounded in a little. Bend your knees and keep feet flat on the floor.

Movement: Gazing at the ceiling, focus on pulling your rib cage and pelvis toward each other. Slowly raise your head and shoulders—not your back—several inches off the floor. Keep your abs flexed. Take seven seconds to crunch up, hold for a second, then take three seconds to lower.

Tips: Your chin shouldn't touch your chest. To keep your head and neck in line, imagine a baseball between your chest and chin. Exhale on the way up; inhale on the way down. Tilt your pelvis to keep your lower back flat on the floor. If you can't get your hand under your back, you're doing it right.

Alternatives: For easier crunches, start with your arms across your chest; gradually work up to hands behind your head. To work the obliques, twist your body side to side as you crunch by aiming your right elbow toward your left knee, then your left elbow toward your right knee. To work the abs in reverse, bring your knee up to your chest so your legs form a 90-degree angle with your body. Bring your knees slightly toward your chest, using only your lower abs.

Your erector spinae runs alongside your spine. The **lower erector spinae**, or **lower back muscles**, straighten your spine. They also work with your abs to stabilize the spine as you move.

Back Extensions (for erector spinae)

Position: Lie on the floor face down with your arms and legs stretched out, your forehead on the floor to keep your neck in line with your back.

Movement: Slowly lift your left arm and right leg several inches. Hold for a second, then slowly lower your arm and leg to your starting position. Repeat with your right arm and left leg. Alternate until you have completed a set.

Tips: Don't arch your back or look up. Pull in your abdominals.

CONTRACT THOSE ABS

In many exercises, you're supposed to tighten (or tense, isolate, flex, pull in) your abs. Why? By flexing your abs, you make sure that they—and not other muscles—do the work. Flexing the abdominals supports your back, stabilizes your trunk, and gives abs an even better workout. How do you contract them? Picture your navel pressing down toward the floor or pulling in toward your spine. You've got it!

inner & outer thighs

Get a leg up on your strength

The muscles of your inner thigh are the **adductors**; your outer thigh muscles are the **abductors**. Adductors pull your legs toward each other. They help you cross your legs, swim the breaststroke, and do jumping jacks. Abductors move your legs out and away from each other. You use them in sports like tennis and golf.

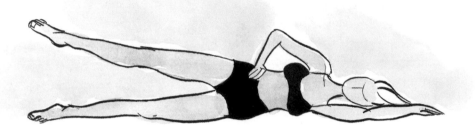

Side Leg Raises (for abductors)

Position: Lie on your left side, head on your extended left arm or on your left elbow. Your right leg should be directly over the left.
Movement: Flex the muscles on the outside of your right thigh and flex your toes as you slowly raise your right leg 12 to 15 inches. Hold for three to five seconds and slowly lower. After completing a set, repeat with the other leg.
Tips: Keep your back still and abs tight.

Side Hip Raises (for abductors)

Position: Stand tall, feet facing forward, three to four inches apart. Hold onto a railing or the back of a chair.
Movement: Slowly raise your right leg directly out to the side (no more than 12 inches high) with your heel leading slightly. Slowly lower. Repeat with the other leg.
Tips: Keep abs tight. Don't lock your knee.

Two muscles, the **gastrocnemius** and the **soleus**, form your calves. They flex your leg at the knee, point your toes, and push off the ground. You use them when you walk, run, jump, bicycle, and tiptoe through the tulips.

Calf Raises (for gastrocnemius)

Position: Stand on a step, feet shoulder-width apart and heels hanging off the edge of the step. For balance, hold onto a rail or a chair, or place your hands against a wall.

Movement: Keeping your legs straight and abs pulled in, raise up on your toes. Flex your calves and hold for a second, then drop your heels until they're slightly lower than the step.

Tip: To maintain balance and posture, pretend you have a string attached to your head that's pulling upward.

EASE INTO IT

For an extra challenge, try adding an ankle weight to your side leg raises and side hip raises.

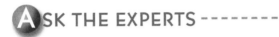

ASK THE EXPERTS

Don't my muscles get enough exercise during my aerobic workout?

Aerobic exercise builds cardiorespiratory and muscle endurance but not muscle strength. What's more, most forms of aerobic exercise do little to build muscle endurance in your upper body.

If I have to stop strength training for a while, will my muscles turn to fat?

Not to worry. Muscles and fat are two different kinds of tissue and can't change from one to the other. If you stop strength training, your muscles will shrink.

buttocks, front thighs, and back thighs

Firm up, no butts about it

The largest muscle in your body, the **gluteus maximus**, or **glute**, is in your buttocks. The gluteus maximus, along with the gluteus medius and gluteus minimus, allows you to extend your hip. They help you walk, stand up, run after your kids, climb stairs, and jump.

The two major muscle groups of your thighs are the **quadriceps**, or **quads**, and **hamstrings**, or—you guessed it—**hams**. Your quads are in the front of your thigh. They straighten your leg from a bent-knee position. You use them to run, walk, stand, ski, and jump. The hams, in the back of your thigh, bend your leg at the knee and help the glutes extend your leg at the hip. They help you stand up, jump, climb stairs, run, or pull your heels up to the backs of your thighs. Working your quads and hams evenly helps prevent knee injury.

Lunges (for glutes, quads, hams)
Position: Stand with your legs together and arms at your sides.
Movement: Step forward two to three feet with your right leg and slowly bend your right knee to lower your body close to the floor, keeping your torso straight and abdominals tight. Keep your right knee directly over your right ankle, with most of your weight on the heel. (You should be able to see your toes.) When your left knee is two inches off the floor, hold for a second. Pushing off with your right foot, return to your starting position. After completing a set, repeat with your left leg.
Tips: You can use a chair for balance. Feel the lunge in your hip and thigh muscles, not in your back, ankles, or knees. For a harder workout, hold a weight in each hand.

Leg Curls (for hams, glutes)

Position: Lie face down on the floor or on a flat bench, legs straight while wearing ankle weights.

Movement: Slowly raise your lower legs until they're perpendicular to the floor, flexing your hamstrings, and slowly lower your legs to the starting position.

Tips: Squeezing your knees together will help you flex your hams. Squeeze your inner thighs together to protect your lower back.

Leg Extensions (for quads)

Position: Sit close to the edge of a chair or a bench while wearing ankle weights. Keep your head up and eyes forward, arms relaxed by your sides.

Movement: Flex your abs and ankles (toes pointed toward the ceiling), and slowly raise your lower legs until they are fully extended. Flex your quads, and slowly return to your starting position.

Tips: Don't lift your thighs. Avoid arching your back.

designing a workout

Muscle fitness is four simple steps away

Here's how to set up an ideal strength-training program.

Step 1. Start a training log. Use a notebook, calendar, or computer.

Step 2. In your log, write the days and times you think you can work out. All you need is 20 minutes, two or three days a week. (Remember to wait at least 48 hours between sessions.)

Step 3. Pick eight to 12 exercises—at least one for each major muscle group—and write them in your log. Be sure to:

- **Work out larger muscles before smaller ones.** If you exercise the smaller muscles first, they'll be too tired to help out when it's time to work larger muscles. Exercise your back and chest before your arms and shoulders. Work your buttocks before your thighs and calves. Don't work your abs too early in the routine; you'll need them to help you exercise other muscles.

BUILDING UP

Within four to six weeks, you should see real progress. If you want to continue building muscle strength, you'll probably need to step up your program every month or two. Remember, the only way to build stronger muscles is to make them work harder. Here's how:

· If you can easily do 12 reps with your current weights, increase the weight by 5 to 10 percent. Lift enough weight so that you struggle through the last rep or two.

· Increase your sets. However, you won't get much benefit from doing more than three sets.

· Choose new exercises to challenge your muscles differently.

· Vary the sequence of exercises. The change in order gives your muscles a different way to work.

Remember that the most noticeable results take place in the first few months. Don't be frustrated if you see less dramatic gains over time.

- **Work out opposing muscle groups in the same session.** For example, your quadriceps oppose your hamstrings: the quads extend your leg and your hamstrings flex it. Other opposing groups are your biceps and triceps, and your abs and lower back. A routine should work groups that oppose each other. Otherwise, one muscle can become stronger than its opposing muscle, increasing the risk of injuring the weaker one.

- **Finish the exercises for one muscle group before moving on.**

Step 4. In your log, note the number of reps and sets you plan to do, and the amount of resistance you'll use. Start with light resistance (three to five pounds per dumbbell) and one set of 10 to 12 reps per exercise.

Voilà! You have a strength-training program!

now what do I do?

Answers to common questions

Q I want a flat stomach. Will strength training do it for me?

Although weight training will strengthen and define muscles, it will not—repeat, will not—help you spot-reduce, no matter what the ads for those best-thing-since-sliced-bread exercise products claim. No machine or exercise can trim fat from one area. The only way you will lose weight (and not just in one spot) is through proper nutrition and aerobic exercise. (Don't forget, strength training helps you burn more calories.) Strength exercises like crunches will make your muscles stronger and look great, but if they're hidden by fat no one will see them.

Q How can I keep up with my strength training when I'm on the road?

Many hotels have excellent gym facilities. If you're used to working with free weights and the hotel gym only has machines, give the machines a try. If your hotel has only free weights, and you've never trained with them, be sure to get instructions on how to use them safely and correctly.

If there are no gym facilities where you're staying, you can always do exercises like push-ups and crunches. Or try working out your muscles by tightening and relaxing them. Here's an example: Stand with one arm by your side, make a fist with it, and flex your biceps. Slowly bend your arm at the elbow, flexing as hard as you can.

You can also pack some resistance in your suitcase. Elastic exercise bands and tubing are a great way to work out when you're on the road. You also can buy a set of water-inflatable dumbbells.

Q Will I look heavier if I lift weights?

No, muscle takes up less space than fat (although it weighs more) so you'll look slimmer, even if your weight stays the same.

BOOKS

Strong Women Stay Slim, Miriam E. Nelson, Ph.D., with Sarah Wernick, Ph.D. A 10-week plan that combines strength training with changes in eating. Includes a food plan with menus and recipes, and illustrated exercises.

Weight Training for Dummies, Liz Neporent and Suzanne Schlosberg Strength-training techniques and exercises, and information on equipment, videos, and classes.

EQUIPMENT

Big Fitness
(800) 383-2008 **www.bigfitness.com**
Weight-training equipment and accessories, and books.

Gym Source
(800) GYM-SOURCE
www.gymsource.com
Free weights, home gyms, accessories, and pre-owned equipment.

VIDEOS

Donna Richardson: 4-Day Rotation Workout
Strength-trains the major muscle groups in 15-minute workouts with dumbbells, including warm-ups and stretches.

Jane Fonda: Total Body Sculpting
Two beginner-intermediate workouts with dumbbells, including warm-ups and cool-downs.

Keys to Weight Training, with Bill Pearl
Techniques and workouts with an emphasis on free weights.

WEB SITES

www.fitnessmagazine.com
Strength-training exercises and workouts, logs, fitness buddies, and how to work out at home.

www.fitnessonline.com
Online group of magazines includes *Shape* (www.shapeonline.com) and *Men's Fitness* (www.mensfitness.com). Strength-training exercises, workouts, and advice.

7

exercising your options

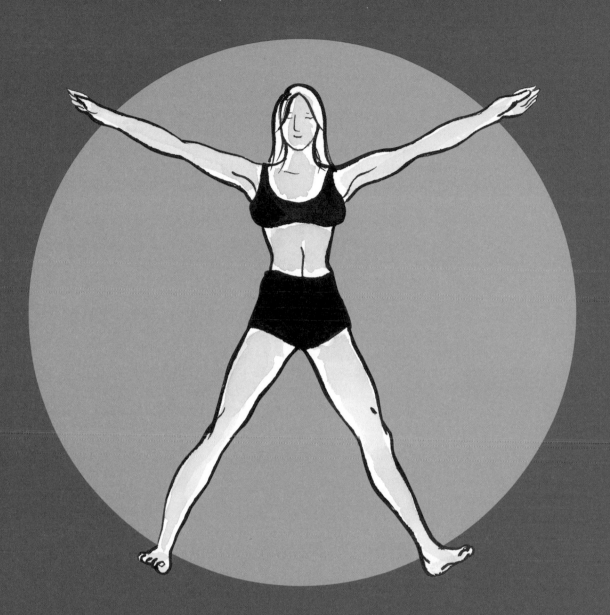

The lowdown on fun exercise from walking
to ski machines, from jumping rope to
swimming. Gone are the days when you say,
"I can't find a single exercise I like."

take your pick

Study the exercise menu

Choosing activities for your fitness program is like ordering a meal in a restaurant. Some selections appeal to you more than others. You can eat chicken piccata each time you visit the restaurant, you can alternate it with grilled tuna, or you can choose something different every time. The key is to pick things that you like. Same goes for choosing an exercise. If you select an activity you don't enjoy, you're less likely to stay the course.

Whatever you choose has to be enjoyable *and* accessible. You can't order strawberry shortcake if strawberries aren't in season, and you won't swim laps if the closest pool is 40 miles away. Your selection must also be affordable. You wouldn't order lobster for dinner—or buy a stairclimber—if you needed the money to pay the rent.

Luckily, there are many selections on the physical activity menu. Choose those that match your current fitness level. If you're just beginning an exercise program or have physical limitations, some activities may be too strenuous. If you have bad knees, for example, a high-impact aerobics class isn't your best choice. If you're overweight, it's better to shed some pounds and take up fitness walking before you run.

This chapter includes many of the most popular aerobic fitness activities. And remember, if you are a beginner, start slowly and gradually build up your activity level. Listen to your body.

So, open up the fitness menu and find what appeals to you, then get ready to design your very own workout program.

EASE INTO IT

Are you looking for a new kind of workout? Call a local gym and ask what classes are offered and when. Pick a class that strikes your fancy and fits into your day. Then make an appointment with yourself to visit the gym and see the class in action.

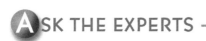

ASK THE EXPERTS

What's high-impact exercise?

High-impact activities require you to take both feet off the ground at the same time. While they strengthen your bones, they're more taxing on your joints. Examples of high-impact activities are running, jogging, jumping rope, and fast-paced aerobics. High-impact activities require a general level of fitness, so wait until you're in better shape to try them.

What's low-impact exercise?

Low-impact activities require that you keep both feet on the ground at all times or shift your weight from one foot to the other. Low-impact exercises include walking, in-line and ice skating, stair-climbing, and slow-paced aerobic dance. If you have joint or lower back pain, or if you're just beginning a fitness program, choose low-impact activities.

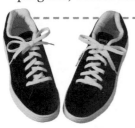

hitting your stride

Put your best foot forward

Nothing's more convenient, or natural, than walking and running. You can walk or run outdoors at the park, a track, the beach, on the street, on a hiking trail, or indoors on a treadmill, at an indoor track, or in the mall. Because they are weight-bearing (you carry your body weight when you do them), walking and running strengthen bones. They also improve your cardiovascular endurance, boost your muscular endurance (especially in your glutes, hamstrings, and quadriceps), and reduce stress. What's more, running and walking won't break the bank: All you need is a pair of good shoes.

Whether you walk or run, follow these tips:
- To warm up and cool down for brisk walking, walk slowly.
- To warm up for running, walk briskly or jog slowly.
- Keep your head and chin up, look straight ahead, relax your shoulders, and pull in your abdominal muscles. Maintain an upright trunk with a slight arch in your lower back, and don't stick out your buttocks.
- Gently cup your hands—as if you're holding a butterfly. Bend your elbows at a 90-degree angle, keeping them close to your sides. When you swing your arms up, don't go higher than your breastbone; on the downswing, brush your hands lightly against your hip.
- Point your feet straight ahead.
- Land on your heel, roll onto your arch, then to the ball of your foot, and push off with your toes.
- To avoid shin splints (painful inflammation of the shin area), walk or run on a more forgiving surface—such as a track, grass, or a dirt path—and follow your workout with the calf stretches in the *Fitness that fits* chapter.
- Don't use hand or ankle weights.
- Wear acrylic or polyester socks to prevent blisters.

Walking is an ideal fitness activity. It puts you at a lower risk of bone and muscle injuries than running, although it burns fewer calories. To walk the walk, take short strides so you don't have to push off so hard with your back foot. Lean forward slightly from your ankles when you're walking at an easy or moderate pace; when you can pick up the pace, lean forward from your hips and slightly from your ankles.

If you're a new fitness walker, start with 10 to 20 minutes. After a month or so, add two or three minutes until you can walk for 30 to 60 minutes. How fast should you walk? Start out slowly and gradually work up to a 12- to 15-minute mile. You'll burn off twice as many calories at that pace as walking a 20-minute mile.

Running provides the benefits of walking and burns more calories than most types of exercise. However, the constant pounding of running is hard on your lower body and can lead to ankle, knee, and hip injuries. It's best to take at least one day off a week from running.

Don't start running until you've walked for a while. Start by alternating a minute of running with a minute of walking for a total of 10 minutes. Do this for two weeks. Then gradually increase the number of minutes you run and decrease your walking time.

FITNESS FACTS

A Footwear Footnote

Invest in a good pair of running or walking shoes. Make sure they absorb shock and have a stable, firm heel counter (the part that wraps around your heel). Walking shoes should be flexible and the heel should be about the same height as the front of the shoe. Running shoes should be flexible at the ball of the foot; and to propel your feet forward, their soles should be about an inch thicker at the heel than at the front of the foot.

A good pair of walking or running shoes should run about $45 to $90. Replace your shoes every 300 to 500 miles, when the tread starts to disappear or the sole wears down.

pedaling to fitness

*Bicycling tips
and gear*

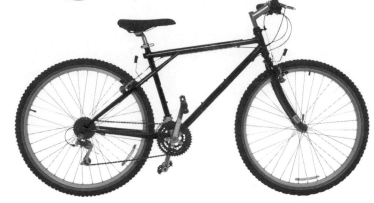

Beautiful scenery, the wind in your hair, your partner right behind you: Bicycling is an enjoyable way to boost cardiovascular fitness, tone and strengthen the muscles in your lower body, and burn lots of calories. It's also easier on your joints than high-impact activities such as running.

Good form will go a long way to prevent neck, knee, and back problems that can plague bicyclists. To prevent knee pain, keep your seat at the right height: your knee should be slightly bent when you push the pedal to its lowest point. Adjust the handlebars so your back isn't stretched out too far, your elbows can bend slightly, and your back isn't any lower than a 50-degree angle to the road. Point your knees straight ahead and pedal all the way through each stroke. (**Toe clips,** straps that hold the front of your shoes, or **clipless pedals** that lock into bicycle cleats, will help you pedal correctly and lower the stress on your knees.) The ball of your foot should line up with the axle of the pedal. Change your hand position on the handlebars frequently. If your knuckles turn white, you're holding on too hard! Warm up and cool down for cycling by riding at an easy pace.

Falls and collisions cause the worst injuries to cyclists. Here are a few tips to keep you safe in the saddle:

- Always wear a helmet—and keep it fastened!
- Use hand signals for turning and stopping.
- Ride on the right-hand side of the road, single file, and in a straight line.
- Brake before you go into a turn.
- Look out for road hazards.

Bicycle Basics

You'll need a chunk of change to buy a bike and accessories—not to mention money for maintenance and repairs. If you want a bicycle that will spend more time on the road than in the repair shop, you'll probably shell out upwards of $250.

The best place to buy a bicycle is a bike shop. Your basic choices are **mountain** (or all-terrain), **road**, or **hybrid** bikes. Mountain bikes, with their wide tires and sturdy frames, are a good choice for cycling off-road or on bad roads. An entry-level mountain bike goes for $250 or so, while performance-type models start around $500. For touring and racing, look for a road bike ($700 plus). It has thinner tires and a lighter frame, but it forces you to hunch over the handlebars. If you're a beginner and plan to ride on a variety of surfaces, a hybrid—a mix of a mountain and a road bike—is a good compromise. It allows you to sit upright (think comfort) and

has sturdier wheels, but it's lighter than a mountain bike and is better suited to riding on pavement. Hybrids start around $300. On a hybrid or road bike, make sure there is one inch between you and the horizontal bar when you straddle the bike, and two or more inches on a mountain bike.

Look for a helmet (about $40) with CPSC certification. (Helmets manufactured in the U.S. after March 1999 must meet this standard.) Make sure it fits snugly. Pick up a pair of padded bike shorts ($40 or so) to cushion your buns and inner thighs, and a gel seat (around $30) to soften the ride. Consider a pair of road gloves to keep your hands from slipping and to absorb shock ($20 and up). Wear shoes with stiff soles. A good pair of bike cleats start around $80. Don't forget a tire-patch kit, a pump, a water bottle, and tools to take along on your rides.

working out, staying in

*Walk, run,
or bike
indoors*

Don't want to brave below-zero temperatures to exercise? Work out in the comfort of your home or at the gym with a treadmill or a stationary bike. These machines deliver a terrific cardio workout and burn lots of calories.

According to the Sporting Goods Manufacturers Association, **treadmills** are the most popular fitness machines in America—for good reason. They're easy to use: all you do is walk or run on a belt. They tone and strengthen your hamstrings, quadriceps, and calves, and put less stress on your lower body than pounding the pavement does.

Expect to pay at least $750 for a quality treadmill. The more expensive models have fancy readouts and preset programs. You're better off with a motorized treadmill, especially if you plan to run on it. Look for one with a two-ply belt and—for durability and to accommodate heavier users—a two horsepower or higher continuous-duty motor. A treadmill with a shock-absorption system is a plus.

Some machines have adjustable inclines for a more strenuous workout. If you're in good shape, look for a treadmill with a 15 percent incline; otherwise, 10 percent is adequate. Plan to run or jog on your treadmill? Buy a machine that reaches 8 to 12 miles per hour. For those occasional stumbles and falls, be sure your treadmill has an automatic on/off switch or a pull cord, and an automatic slow-start feature. (Never step on a treadmill unless you're sure it's not on and not moving fast.)

A few treadmill tips: Be sure to pick up your feet and look straight ahead when you run or walk. You'll get a better workout by swinging your arms, but if you need the handrails for balance, hold on lightly and don't lean back. And as much as you might feel like it, don't drape yourself over the console!

Indoor cycling is another way to kick your workout into high gear. Buy a **wind trainer** (a piece of equipment that your outdoor bike sits on while you pedal) for under $100, or hop on a stationary bike. Expect to pay around $400 for a basic bike and up to $3,000 for one with preset programs and elaborate readouts. Some bikes are upright; others are recumbent. **Upright bikes** target your quadriceps, buttocks, and hips; some have attachments to work your arms. On an upright bike, the key is to sit up straight so you don't stress your neck and back. **Recumbent bikes**, which support your lower back as you pedal out in front of you, target your buns and hamstrings. With both types of stationary bikes, you can change the resistance to intensify the workout.

Be sure to adjust the seat so your knee is slightly bent when the pedal is at its lowest point. Warm up and cool down by riding the bike slowly, walking briskly, or jogging. Start out slowly: cycle for 12 to 15 minutes using low resistance for the first month. Gradually up your workout by cycling longer and adding resistance.

stepping it up

Shape up with stairclimbers and elliptical trainers

Looking for a different kind of aerobic exercise? Stairclimbers and elliptical trainers may be right up your alley. Sure, you could climb the steps at home or at the office for exercise. But climbing real steps can do a number on your knees. Stairclimbers provide a low-impact workout that's easier on your knees than hiking up and down your basement stairs. It's also easier on your neck and back than cycling. You'll tone your buns and quadriceps, and because stairclimbing is a weight-bearing activity, you'll also strengthen your bones.

Stairclimbers come in two varieties. One is a **rolling staircase**, which is like an escalator. The other is sometimes called a **stepper**. You stand on two foot plates and press down with one foot while you pick up the other foot. The rolling climber is more strenuous because the level of the step is set; you can't cheat by taking baby steps like you might do on a stepper. Both types of equipment have adjustable resistance and speed.

Stairclimbers can tire out your legs, so they may be too intense if you're not in good shape. You also may experience pain if you have knee or hip problems.

FITNESS FACTS

Ladder-Climbing Machines

No, that guy in the gym isn't climbing up a ladder to change a light bulb. He's on a **ladder-climbing machine**. This machine, with its long, vertical stick and pedals, delivers a low-impact upper- and lower-body workout. You can step, walk, jog, or climb on it: Just adjust the tension and the speed, and you're off. You can use this machine in a gym or purchase one (for about $1400) for your home.

Wear flexible shoes, such as cross-trainers. Warm up and cool down by climbing at a slow speed. Stand up straight but lean forward slightly at your hips so you don't lock your knees or strain your lower back. Keep your abdominals pulled in to support your back. Fight the temptation to lean on the handrails. On a stepper, put your entire foot on the pedal and press through your heel. Pace your steps so they're fairly deep and even.

Stairclimbers are expensive: A quality machine will run at least $1,500. If you're in the market for the stepper variety, you'll get a better workout with a machine whose steps move independently of each other.

Elliptical trainers are one of the latest entries to the fitness world. These machines combine the movements of a stairclimber, a cross-country ski machine, and a treadmill. You put your feet on the pedals and move them either forward or backward in an elongated circular motion, changing the intensity of the workout by adjusting speed, incline, and resistance. Elliptical trainers work your lower body, especially your quadriceps. They're also easier on knees than stairclimbers. An elliptical trainer costs anywhere from $1,800 to $3,000.

moving in sync

Step, kick, cycle, and spin

If you enjoy working out with other people, prefer a structured workout, or need some extra motivation, **aerobics classes** may be right for you. These classes improve cardiovascular endurance, coordination, balance, flexibility, and muscle strength and endurance, while helping burn calories. Whether the class is low-impact, high-impact, hip-hop, slide, circuit, studio cycling, kick-boxing, interval, or step, an instructor typically leads the group through a 45- to 60-minute session of aerobic exercises choreographed to music. If you prefer to work out at home, throw an aerobics video into the VCR and get moving!

A typical class includes a warm-up, light stretches, an aerobic portion, cool-down, and more stretches. Usually, gyms offer several levels of classes, from beginner to advanced. If you're just starting to get in shape, go for a beginner class and stay away from high-impact sessions. To lower the stress on your body, be sure to work out on a wood or densely carpeted floor. Wear comfortable clothes and a good pair of either aerobics or cross-training shoes with lots of cushioning and support (less than $80 or so).

If you feel like stepping to the music, try a **step aerobics** class. These classes help strengthen and tone your buns and legs. You step on and off a platform about two or three feet long that rests on the floor or atop one or more risers. Once you learn the basic moves—getting on and off the platform, over, and across it—an instructor leads you through a routine. A few downsides: Excessive step aerobics can lead to knee or lower-back problems, and it takes a bit of coordination to get the hang of the moves. Wear either special step shoes or aerobics shoes. If you'd rather work out at home, buy a step system (around $75) and work out with a video.

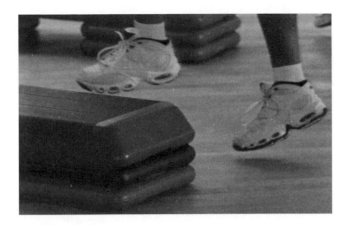

Here are a few stepping tips:
- If you're a beginner, start with a platform height of 4 to 6 inches. Don't worry about the arm movements until you've got the steps down.
- The height of the step shouldn't make you bend your knees more than 90 degrees.
- Keep your neck straight, shoulders back, pelvis tucked, abdominals pulled in, chest lifted, and don't arch your back.
- When stepping onto the platform, lean from your ankles.
- Place your whole foot on the platform so it doesn't tip.
- Don't pound when you step.

Do you avoid exercise classes because you don't want to keep up with the pack? One of the latest fitness rages, **studio cycling** (also called **spinning** and **indoor cycling**) lets you control the intensity and pace of a workout while you enjoy the motivation of group exercise. In these classes, the instructor leads the class on an imaginary ride that includes hills, which you simulate by increasing the resistance on the bike. It's a more strenuous workout than outdoor cycling, so don't try it unless you're in reasonably good shape.

jumping and skating

Don't skip jumping rope and in-line skating

Do you want to feel like a kid again? Try jumping rope and in-line skating. **Jumping rope** has a lot going for it. It's inexpensive and you can jump anywhere—throw a rope into your suitcase and keep up with your workouts on the road. Jumping rope works your cardiorespiratory system and improves agility as well as hand and foot coordination. What's more, it firms your shoulder, arm, and leg muscles. It helps build bones and burns more calories, minute for minute, than just about any activity.

Because jumping rope is so intense, it's difficult to keep it up for more than 5 to 10 minutes. Make this activity part of your routine, mixing it up with something like a treadmill or a stationary bike.

The best way to jump is only an inch or so—just high enough to clear the rope. This makes the workout less stressful on your knees and ankles.

Here are a few pointers:
- Grip the handles lightly and turn the rope from your wrists, keeping hands at waist level and elbows close to your body.
- Jump on a shock-absorbing surface, such as a rubber mat or a wood floor.
- Keep your knees slightly bent.
- Keep your back straight, abdominals pulled in, and head up.

To start, mix 15 to 20 seconds of jumping with 30 to 40 seconds of walking in place or resting. Gradually, up the jumping time and decrease rest periods.

Ropes have come a long way from the clothesline variety of your youth. Many are made of synthetic materials; some have weighted handles. They sell for about $4 and up, depending on the material and the features. Look for a lightweight rope with foam grips, which will keep your hands from slipping when they sweat. To determine if a rope is the right length, step on the center of it with one foot. The handles should come up to your armpits. As for footwear, aerobics or cross-training shoes are fine, as long as they provide cushioning for the ball of your foot (where you'll land) and adequate support.

Looking for a fun alternative to walking and running? **In-line skating**, also called **blading**, gives you a great low-impact cardio workout, improves balance and coordination, strengthens the muscles in your lower back, hips and legs, and burns lots of calories.

Consider renting skates before buying them, as you'll pay upwards of $100 for a pair. A word of caution: In-line skaters suffer their share of wipeouts. The most common injuries are to arms, wrists, and hands. Be sure to use wrist guards, elbow and knee pads ($25 to $50 for a set of all three), and always wear a helmet that protects the back of your head (a biking helmet is OK). It's well worth the cost to take a few lessons; you need to learn to stop, control your speed, turn, and deal with road hazards.

Warm up and cool down by skating slowly. To skate properly, bend your knees and lean forward slightly. If you feel a fall coming on, don't stand up or lean back; instead, bend forward and reach for your knees. When you know you're going to fall, try to drop to your knees.

pooling your assets

Dive into swimming and water aerobics

So, you don't like to perspire when you work out? No sweat. **Swimming** or **water exercise** (also called **aquatics**, **aquacize**, or **aqua aerobics**) could be for you. You'll improve cardiovascular fitness and flexibility, build muscular strength and endurance, and burn calories. Unlike many other activities, water workouts exercise both the upper and lower body. But because of the buoyancy of the water, water exercise doesn't stress your joints the way other activities, such as running, do. If you're overweight or recovering from an injury, swimming is an ideal exercise.

To warm up and cool down for lap swimming, swim at an easy pace. If you're a beginner, aim to swim four laps in a 25-meter pool, resting one minute between laps (the length of the pool and back). Over time, increase the number of laps you can do without stopping. Although you're most likely to swim the **front crawl**, also called **freestyle**, throw in some other strokes, such as the **breaststroke** and the **backstroke**, to work different muscle groups.

Swimmers may suffer from overuse injuries and pulled muscles. Learning the right technique will help you avoid injuries. Aim for big and slow strokes, and kick from your hips. For safety, be sure to swim where there is a lifeguard.

Water exercise equipment won't sink your wallet. Buy a good pair of goggles to protect your eyes from chlorine and help you see better underwater ($10 and up). Hand paddles (around $15), webbed gloves ($10 to $15), and water dumbbells ($20-$30) increase resistance to give you a more intense upper-body workout. Holding onto a kickboard ($10 to $15) helps you concentrate on kicking.

Flotation belts ($10 to $30) and vests ($40 and up) make it easier to work out in deep water.

If group workouts whet your appetite, find an aqua exercise class. To exercise on your own, try walking or running in waist-deep water, or treading water.

designing your workout

*Time to put
it all together*

Now that you understand the three components of a solid fitness program—aerobic fitness, strength training, and stretching—you can incorporate them into a program that fits your needs. If you're new to exercise, or you've taken off a while, start slowly and comfortably, and work your way up. Allow your body to adjust to the workload.

At the beginning, focus on frequency and time. Don't worry about boosting intensity until you've consistently marshaled 30 minutes a day, three days a week. If you're too out of breath to carry on a conversation, you're working too hard and need to slow down.

For your aerobics exercises, warm up for about five minutes, then slowly increase the load or pick up the pace until you reach your target heart zone. For the first four to six weeks, make this zone 40 to 60 percent of your maximum heart rate and sustain it for 12 to 15 minutes, if you can. Keep moving in some way or other for 10 minutes more. Gradually lengthen the time you work out. As you get in better shape, you'll want to be able to maintain 55 to 85 percent of your maximum heart rate for 20 to 60 minutes. The higher the intensity, the shorter the workout needs to be (no less than 20 minutes, though) to reap similar cardiovascular benefits.

Cool down for about five minutes, slowing your pace or decreasing the load until your body returns to a resting level. Then, stretch the muscles you used during the workout for at least three minutes.

Strength-train your major muscle groups (arms, chest, shoulders, abs, back, buttocks, thighs, and calves) two to three days a week. To review, use a weight you can lift at least 10 times, but no more than 12 times, without fatigue. Don't skip this part! If you don't build muscle, you lose it, no matter how many aerobics classes you take in a week!

Finally, incorporate stretching into your routine. (See pages 114-119). All you need is at least 10 minutes a day, at least two or three times a week—a tiny investment considering the overwhelming returns: improved athletic performance and range of motion, not to mention injury prevention.

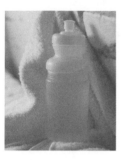

After a while, your body will get used to the workload. Once you adjust to the exertion, you'll stay fit but won't improve much more. To continue to make headway, you need to work your body harder than it's used to. Increase your frequency, intensity, or time spent working out. If you go a little harder each week, you can continue to improve without spending more time working out. If you want to lose weight and boost your cardio endurance, increase both the frequency and duration of your workouts.

FITNESS FACTS

Once you get used to working out, spice things up to avoid boredom and to fine-tune your conditioning. Try these exercise variations:

Cross-train. To get out of a rut, work your muscles differently, and help reduce the risk of overuse injuries, integrate more than one exercise into your routine. Instead of jogging every day, for example, bike one day, row the next, and jog another. For strength training, you could work with free weights one day, rock-climb another day, and hit the machines at the gym the next time.

Interval-train. To jack up your power—to get a good first step toward the tennis net, for example—incorporate bursts of intense exertion into your workout. If you normally jog, run for a minute or two; if you usually swim leisurely laps, sprint for a lap or two. Resume your normal pace and allow your body to level off, then go back to the bursts.

Circuit-train. To accomplish strength and conditioning work at the same time, move from one exercise to the next without stopping. Fill time between your weight sets with a couple of minutes of an aerobic activity. You might opt for the stationary bike, jump rope, or row. When you're finished, you've completed both aerobics and strength-training requirements at the same time!

now what do I do?

Answers to common questions

Q How can I stop getting a stitch in my side when I exercise?

A side stitch is a message from your body to slow down. One cause of these side aches is eating too much, or too soon, before you exercise. Another cause may be weak stomach muscles. If you have a side stitch, slow down your activity level until you feel better. Also, try using stomach muscles to breathe more deeply. If the side aches persist, seek medical attention.

Q What's the difference between running and jogging?

The difference between jogging and running is the pace. Jogging is simply running at a slower speed.

Q Do I get enough exercise when I play touch football on the weekends?

Playing a sport can improve muscle tone and coordination, relieve stress, and burn calories. But if it isn't continuous and sustained—you stop and start—you may not be getting enough of a cardiorespiratory workout.

Q What activity can I do to build muscle strength and endurance in my major muscle groups?

Give a rowing machine a try. It improves cardiovascular fitness and increases flexibility and mobility. And, since it's non-impact, it's easy on your joints. Warm up and cool down by rowing slowly. If you're a beginner, row for 10 to 15 minutes at a slow pace. Work up to 15 to 30 rows per minute. Keep your body relaxed and don't jerk. Let your legs and buttocks—not your back—power the early part of the rowing motion. Be careful not to lock your knees or hunch over. If you're in the market for a rowing machine, look for one with a flywheel mechanism. Expect to spend between $700 and $800.

BOOKS

Fitness Aquatics, LeAnne Case
Tips on getting started, equipment, and 60 workouts in levels based on duration and length.

Workouts for Dummies, Tamilee Webb, M.A., with Lori Seeger, M.A.
Tips for designing a workout that matches your body type and goals. Advice for workouts at home, in the gym, at work, or on the road. Sections for children, pregnant women, and older adults.

The Beginning Runner's Handbook: The Proven 13-Week Walk/Run Program, Ian MacNeill and the Sports Medicine Council of British Columbia
A plan to ease into running, with advice and motivation.

EQUIPMENT

AquaJogger
(800) 922-9544
www.aquajogger.com
Buoyancy belts, webbed gloves, weights, resistance footwear, and videos for water workouts.

Beyond Moseying
(800) 490-2800
www.beyondmoseying.com
Treadmills, stationary bikes, elliptical trainers, steppers, ladder-climbing machines, rowers, and strength-training equipment.

MAGAZINES

Runner's World
(800) 666-2828
www.runnersworld.com

VIDEOS

Linda Evans' The New You, with Kari Anderson
Beginner-intermediate. Features three progressively challenging segments with music by Yanni and tips on diet, fitness, and motivation.

Kathy Smith's Latin Rhythm Workout
Cardio workout through Latin dancing. Includes instruction on partner dancing.

8

maintaining ever after

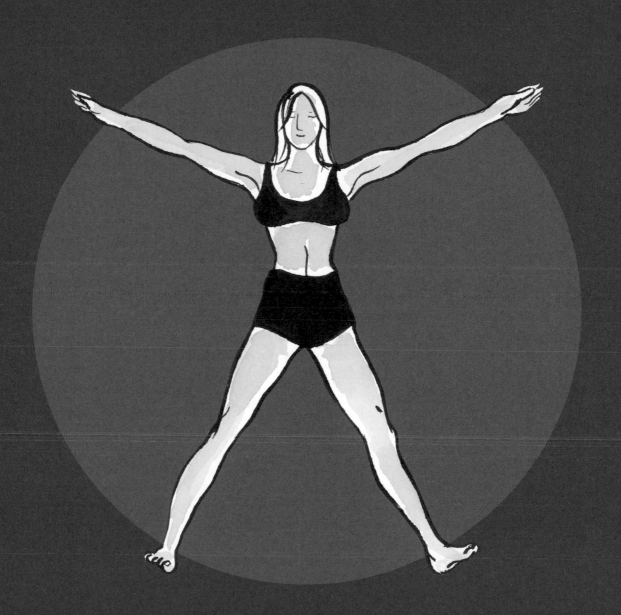

Kudos—you're in shape! But what about
maintaining the new, healthier you?
How do you deal with eating out, going on
the road, and other real-life events?
Read on and see how.

making exercise work out

Sticking with the program

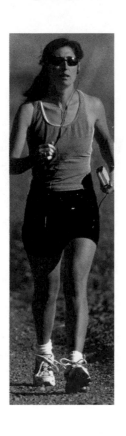

Okay, you know which exercises you're supposed to do and how you're supposed to do them. How do you stick with an exercise program? That's where things can get a little tricky. Well-intentioned exercisers abandon their fitness quests for all sorts of reasons, from injuries to inconvenience to just plain boredom. But a few maintenance steps can prevent this, setting the stage for a lifetime of success.

When you start exercising regularly, the pounds and fat seem to melt away and your endurance makes major strides. But after a while, you get so fit that the results aren't obvious. That's when you might start to stutter. You can fend off this peril by cross training. For example, instead of affixing yourself to the stair climber each workout, do different exercises on different days. Hike, bike, run, swim, climb rocks, row, ski, skate, spin, kick-box, or play hockey, basketball, or soccer. This will infuse your workouts, body, and mind with a new challenge and a sense of adventure. It's less stressful on your body than hard, repetitive movements, and you get a better workout because you are using different muscles.

Working out is something to look forward to—an invigorating, satisfying release. If you don't enjoy your workouts, you're either trying to exercise at the wrong time or you're doing the wrong exercise. Change the time, the location, the machine—even the exercise itself. Try new sports, videotapes, and techniques until you find something you truly enjoy. Be careful not to drop your whole program while you search for something new. Keep up your aerobic activity while you experiment. To eliminate workout boredom, listen to your favorite music or audiobook, watch TV, hook up with a buddy, take a class—do whatever you can to keep things fun.

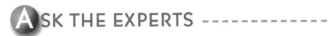

ASK THE EXPERTS

Some days I'm just plain tired and can't imagine running for 40 minutes on the treadmill. Any suggestions?

When you feel too tired to get started, you might simply be out of energy. Eat a little something. Have a bagel, a banana, or a hard-boiled egg. (Nothing heavy.) If you know lack of food isn't the problem, just take a walk outside or a saunter on the treadmill. You might be surprised at how quickly you perk up! If you don't, no sweat. Every single workout session won't be perfect. The important thing is to keep moving, and to keep your commitment to a workout time. If you're always tired, you might want to consider changing your workout time.

I hurt my elbow and my doctor says it will take six weeks to recover. Do I have to stop everything while I wait?

With many injuries there's no reason to stop exercising altogether. Simply switch to an exercise that doesn't stress the injured part of your body (like walking if your upper body is injured or, for certain lower-body injuries, swimming.) If you're unsure what to do, ask your doctor, a physical therapist, or a personal trainer.

keeping the family fit

Making exercise child's play

By shaping up you have taken the first step toward helping your loved ones get in shape! Experts say the apple doesn't fall far from the tree when it comes to fitness. In other words, if you park yourself in front of the computer or TV and order your kids outside, they won't get it. They emulate what you do. Turn off the electronics and go out with them.

Why bother? You rescue your kids from becoming part of an alarming statistic—nearly one in four is overweight, twice as many as 30 years ago. You can help spare them now from poor health, lack of energy, and ridicule.

Turn getting fit into family fun. Schedule a time to shape up together and stick to it. Choose activities appropriate to your family members' ages, interests, and fitness levels. To keep things engaging, have a different family member choose the activity each week.

You might not all be able to bike or play tennis together, but you can probably all hike together. Depending on the ages of your kids, hoola-hoop; play hopscotch, Frisbee or tennis; have a long-jump tournament; wash the car together; shoot hoops; swim at the rec center; build stilts and strut on them; run through the sprinkler; bowl; hang on the monkey bars; or play Twister. Take lessons in fun activities like juggling or kite flying, in-line skating, snowshoeing, karate, or golf.

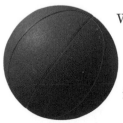

With your partner, change the nature of your time together. Instead of dinner and the movies, for example, have a light picnic in the park and go dancing or bowling. Bike or hike a scenic route, walk the beach, or go dancing. Slowly incorporate more activity as your family becomes fit.

I was so excited one day when my kids agreed to go jogging with me at the high school track. I was glad they joined me. But when it came time to run, my 12-year-old couldn't make it half a mile and my 8-year-old kept lagging behind to study bugs. I was frustrated because I couldn't get in a workout, and my kids demaned to go home.

So much for fit and fun time! A couple of days later my husband took them to the pool. I imagined a disaster but they all came back smiling. They played water tag and had races. My husband used a kickboard while the kids swam freestyle. He adapted his workout to their level—not theirs to his.

—Stacey R., Ames, Iowa

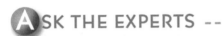SK THE EXPERTS

I explain to my teenage daughter how important it is to get fit, and I keep inviting her to join me on my walks. But you know what it's like talking to teenagers. Half the time all I get out of her is a grunt. What can I do?

Even if she doesn't want to be seen outside with you, there's hope indoors. Invite a personal trainer to your home, or set up a spot where you both can strength-train or do aerobics. Work out on your own schedules, but commit to exercising together at least once a week. Let her choose the time and the music. Exercise may boost her self-esteem, elevate her mood, make her feel strong, peaceful, coordinated, and flexible. Before you know it, you might even have a conversation.

feeding your family

Getting the kids juiced for fruits and veggies

Time to call a family meeting, one of those powwows that always seemed to work for the Brady Bunch. The issue at hand: your family's diet. The motivation: developing good eating habits for your family now to keep them healthy and protect them from the battle of the bulge later.

Explain that you are so excited by the prospect of everyone feeling healthy and energetic that you are all going to eat healthfully at home. Ask your family to help banish from the house foods that do everyone in: junk food in the cabinets, buckets of fried chicken, mountains of fries, or leaning towers of pizza—they're all out (except for the occasional splurge; you don't want to totally freak out the kids).

This is an important event, so be prepared. Have on hand tasty, good-for-you snacks—fruit salad, spiced popcorn, healthy muffins and breads, or whatever you think they might enjoy. Share recipes you know will appeal to your family and encourage them to choose those they'd like to try. Show them that this quest will be fun, enjoyable, and delicious.

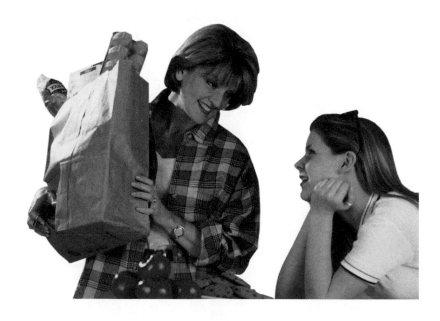

Will everyone share your enthusiasm? Fat chance. They'll probably be skeptical at best, complaining at worst. Keep things low key at first. Simply power up the usual fare. Stir some silky-style tofu into macaroni and cheese to boost protein. Mix a healthier look-alike into the kids' favorite sugary cereal. Add a few teaspoons of non-fat dry milk to meatloaf, pancakes, or muffins to boost calcium. Mix exotic fruits into frosties in the blender. Puree carrots or zucchini in the food processor and add them to spaghetti sauce, meatloaf, or burgers.

Remain positive and keep the healthful foods coming. Eventually, everyone will come around.

FITNESS FACTS

Relax When It Comes to Snacks

Snacks aren't evil. In fact, the right snacks can help your family's shape-up efforts. If your kids are young, offer snacks from the food groups they are short on that day: perhaps sliced fruit; broccoli; carrot, celery, or cucumber sticks; low-fat cheese and crackers; or cereal and yogurt for a grain and protein combo. Offer a snack before the kids become ravenous and won't settle for anything other than cookies. Resist the temptation to park the food and the kids in front of the TV—this quickly becomes another bad habit.

For your teens, yourself, and your mate, keep low-fat cheese, veggies, and fruits that are already peeled and cut in the fridge—perfect to grab and go. Teach your teens how to microwave a potato and crown it with quick, easy toppings like low-fat mozzarella and tomato sauce for a pizza potato, or salsa and low-fat Monterey Jack cheese for a Mexican potato. You also can put these toppings on whole grain pitas, bagels, or English muffins.

Ask family members not to bring you or your kids bags of candy and cookies. If this is simply too outrageous a thought, graciously accept the sweets —then either toss them out after Grandma leaves or share them at the office.

It's okay to bend the rule on holidays, but always have healthful options on hand.

eating out

Dining tips made to order

Some days it is impossible to eat at home. Work consumes the hours, family members scatter, the fridge stands bare. Other days, eating out is a cherished time to relax, socialize, celebrate, eat something that tastes great, get served, and have someone else clean up. Whatever the reason, the average American eats out four times a week—and probably has an expanded waistline to show for it.

Eating out can wreak havoc on your shape-up efforts, but it doesn't have to if you follow some simple strategies.

Before you leave for a restaurant, drink a couple of glasses of water and eat some fresh fruit or veggies. Otherwise, by the time you get there you could be so hungry you'll want to eat not only the bread and butter at the table, but the basket, too. To help control what you eat, carefully choose where you eat. Will you go to a place that serves French fries? Or one that serves fruit cups? Fried chicken or fajitas? Head for a restaurant that serves a variety of tasty, healthful fare.

Once you get there, don't be afraid to specify what you want. If you'd rather have steamed vegetables than those sauteed in butter, say so. If you prefer pasta in tomato sauce rather than in cream, request it. If you prefer shrimp broiled or grilled, not fried, just ask. Chefs are often happy to accommodate special requests.

Beware of hidden fats. At a restaurant, you can't read nutrition labels to find out what's in a dish, so you have to do some investigating. (If the waiter doesn't know, politely request that he check with the chef.) Is the broccoli soup cream- or vegetable-based? Is the grilled chicken marinated in oil? Is there butter and cream in the mashed potatoes?

Size up the servings. The USDA says a portion of meat is three ounces. The Saturday night special Slab o' Beef could tip the scales at a pound or more! If the restaurant serves large portions, ask the waiter ahead of time to serve you half and to wrap the rest for you to take home. If you decide to eat the whole thing anyway, at least substitute a salad or a baked potato (no butter) for the fries.

Don't drink alcohol before your food arrives. It fills you with empty calories and decreases willpower. Instead, drink water, sparkling water, club soda, or if you must, diet soda, and send back the basket of nacho chips or bread and butter at the table.

Beware of the salad bar, where diet-killing demons can attack unsuspecting dieters. If a vegetable looks glossy, it's probably covered in fatty oil. Three-bean salad, marinated mushrooms, pasta salad—they might pack more fat and calories than a giant burger with fries! Bypass chunks of cheese, croutons, bacon, and anything mayonnaisy, like potato or tuna salad. Choose dressing that's low-fat or fat-free, or dress your salad with lemon juice or vinegar.

If you want to splurge, decide ahead of time during which part of the meal you will do it, then amend the rest of your order accordingly. For example, if the Italian restaurant has the greatest *tiramisu* for dessert and you plan on eating it, don't get cheesy garlic bread for an appetizer, or lasagna for your entrée. On the other hand, if you're going for a fat-filled entrée, order a lean vegetable dish or salad with low-fat dressing and skip the dessert (or share one with a friend).

Most importantly, **enjoy yourself.** Don't ruin a meal by feeling guilty as you eat. If you overdo it, simply make changes during the week and get back on track.

Tips Made-to-Order

Chinese

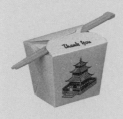

Don't eat the fried noodles on the table. They're loaded with fat. Instead, take the edge off your hunger with wonton, egg drop, or hot and sour soup. Stay away from anything called crispy, fried, or deep-fried. Opt for steamed, roasted, or stir-fried dishes (request that your order be cooked with as little oil as possible). If you don't know how something is made, ask. Load up on nutrients with steamed vegetables and brown rice. If you haven't already tried tofu (also called bean curd), this is a great place to try it. Chinese restaurants tend to offer a terrific assortment of tofu dishes.

Mexican

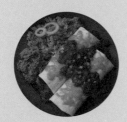

Again, stay away from the chips and avoid anything with a fried, crispy shell. (This includes chimichangas, tostadas, flautas, and hard tacos. If something you want is served in a fried shell, ask if the chef can serve it in a soft tortilla instead, or with soft tortillas on the side.) Go easy on the cheese, sour cream, and guacamole. Help yourself to gazpacho or ask for jicama and salsa. Fajitas, burritos, grilled meats, and fish are excellent entrée choices.

Italian

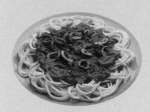

Skip the fried mozzarella, and order soup or salad first. Avoid anything parmigiana (often fried, then smothered with cheese), pastas stuffed with cheese or sausage, and anything in a cream sauce. Opt for red sauce or wine sauce, or select roasted or grilled fish and meats. If you order scampi, ask them to go easy on the oil or butter. For pizza, go with a thin crust, topped with vegetables and sprinkled with cheese. Or try something different on top—instead of mountains of mozzarella, sausage, or olives, get adventurous with combinations such as clams and spinach with a sprinkling of parmesan, or grilled chicken and red peppers with feta scattered on top.

Deli

Given the choice of what to sandwich between their bread—roast beef or a salad of tuna, chicken, or turkey—many people believe they're better off calorie- and fat-wise if they don't pick the beef. But the salads pack loads of hidden calories and fat because of the mayonnaise. Mayonnaise can undermine your best efforts. Just one tablespoon contains 100 calories—all of them from fat. That's already 17 percent of your total fat for the day! So skip the salads (including mayonnaise-filled macaroni and potato salad and coleslaw). If you order a meat-filled sandwich, don't add mayo or butter. If you're at one of those delis that overstuffs sandwiches, buy a plain roll, take half the meat out of the sandwich, and make yourself another one for tomorrow's breakfast or lunch. And bag the corn or potato chips. If you want something crunchy on the side, go with pretzels or, better yet, carrot sticks.

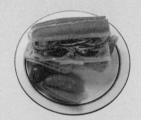

Fast Food

If it's one of those days when the drive-thru at Burger Buddies seems unavoidable, skip the mayo or "special sauce," avoid salad dressing and cheese, and don't get anything fried (even chicken and fish are not healthy choices when fried). Instead, order grilled chicken or a burger (not supersized) with mustard or ketchup, or a baked potato. If you're temporarily beyond reason and you must get fries, order the regular size or share your order. If you're going for fast tacos, avoid waist-busters like taco salad with dressing in an edible shell, which packs more calories and fat than a personal pan pepperoni pizza, or a megaburger with special sauce! Wherever and whatever you order, try to salvage the meal by ordering skim milk instead of soda. (Soda has twice as many calories and negligible nutrients.) If you have time, bring along some cut-up fruits and veggies for you and the kids to eat on the way.

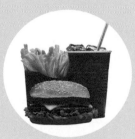

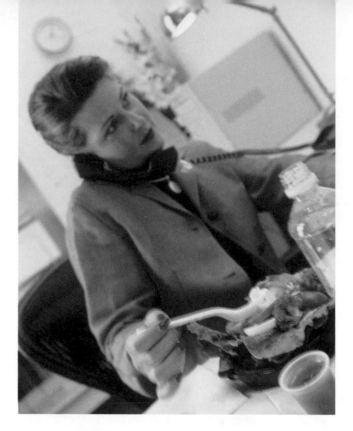

staying fit on the job

When working in keeps you from working out

Even with the best intentions, many days you just can't squeeze in a trip to the gym during lunchtime, or meetings interrupt your before- or after-work exercise routine. Too often, these stumbling blocks can derail your shape-up program.

But work doesn't have to thwart your fitness quest. Simply change your mindset to include working in movement on the job when you can. Moving will clear your mind as well as help you get fit.

When the day's workout doesn't seem possible, leave for work a few minutes early and park the car farther from the building or the train. While on the job, take five minutes each hour and move your body: Walk to the next floor to use the water cooler or the restroom. (Don't cheat and use the elevator.) Stretch different parts of your body, from raising your eyebrows to wiggling your toes. Deliver your messages to colleagues in the same building instead of phoning or e-mailing them. Put a twist on your breaks: Walk around the parking lot, the building, the neighborhood, or the parking garage for 15 or 20 minutes—whatever you can spare. No amount of time is too little. Before you get in the car to go home, take a 15-minute walk.

Try to find colleagues who share your desire to shape up and agree to have your meetings outside and talk while you walk. Start a campaign to have the company hook up with a fitness center or provide space or equipment on-site where you can all exercise.

FITNESS FACTS

Working It

If you have your own office, you're really in luck. Not because you can close the door and play solitaire for hours on end, but because you can turn your work space into your workout space. Need to get the creative juices flowing? Close the door and crank out some push-ups, sit-ups, leg lifts and raises, back extensions, lunges, and calf raises. Keep weights in your file cabinets so you can work on your bicep curls while you deal with your most annoying client on the speakerphone. Follow up with your triceps, delts, pecs, and lats.

If you don't have your own office, not to worry. You can do leg lifts and crunches from your chair in your cubicle, standing push-ups against a wall in the bathroom, and lunges in the elevator. No one will notice a thing—except how fit you're beginning to look!

on the road

*Pack ahead—
or pack 'em on*

Even when you manage to work out around work, the inevitable happens—work or a getaway takes you on the road. Nothing like a little jaunt to trip up your shape-up plans: Bacon for breakfast, lobster for lunch, duck for dinner. Who wants to exercise when conference sessions end, considering the fun that awaits at happy hour?

Putting your workouts on hold while you travel can sidetrack you on your road to fitness. Once you lose the rhythm of your workout routines it can be hard to get it back. Don't give up. Instead, devise a health strategy before you hit the road. Call around and reserve

---

FITNESS FACTS

Just Plane Smart

When you reserve your plane ticket, ask about meal options. At no extra cost, you can request low-fat and low-sodium meals, among other alternatives to the standard fare. If food won't be served on board, bring along the makings of a quick, healthy snack: pretzels, carrot sticks, a banana, or apple. Or pack dried fruit and a cereal bar. They're easy to carry, don't have to be kept cold, won't squish like fresh fruit, and don't need preparation.

Flying is dehydrating. Be sure to bring a bottle of water; drink it down in the airport, and refill it for the flight. While in flight, stay away from coffee, tea, and alcohol, all of which dehydrate you even more. Instead, ask for water or vegetable juice to hydrate you and boost your daily liquid nutrients.

a room where there's a pool or fitness center on-site. Find out what equipment the center offers, the busiest workout times (so you can avoid them), and other fitness options the hotel provides, such as maps of walking or running routes in the neighborhood, or a free pass at a local fitness center. If the hotel offers in-room VCRs, bring along a couple of fitness tapes, and complement them with hotel room-friendly exercises such as push-ups, sit-ups, curls, jumping jacks, and isometrics.

Pack for working out. Toss a jump rope in your suitcase, bring along plastic dumbbells that you can fill with water later to add weight. Pack a bathing suit, shorts, and T-shirts. Put your sneakers in your carry-on bag so you can take a brisk walk if the opportunity arises during your journey.

Remember to eat smart, using the tips for eating out that you learned earlier in this chapter.

staying in shape

Taking the routine out of your routine

If you want your new healthy lifestyle to work for good, you need to reshape your habits. You don't need to undergo any major renovations—just tweak things a bit as you go along and seize easy fitness opportunities each day.

For example, approach chores differently by making them mini-aerobics sessions. Vacuum, scrub, sweep, or wash your car double time, with your favorite music blasting. In the grocery store, stride up and down the aisles. Instead of putting your dog out in the yard, take him for a walk. Walk or bike with your kids to school or to the bus stop. At the store, park in a space that's a hike from the entrance. Walk the escalator rather than riding it. Better yet, take the stairs—and if you can, take them two at a time (hold onto the rail!). Instead of paying someone to mow your lawn, do it yourself. Working in the yard, cleaning, and washing the windows give the house—and you—visible results.

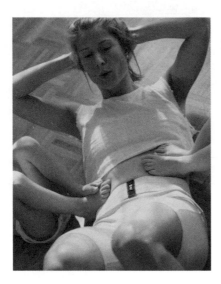

Get down and dirty in the garden. When you talk on the phone, pace the floor or stretch your muscles. When you watch TV, lift weights, stretch, or do some strength training like crunches or push-ups. Get the kids in the act, too.

To fuel your enthusiasm and school your technique, subscribe to a fitness or healthful cooking magazine, or ask for a gift subscription. Try a new sport or take a cooking class.

When Your Efforts Lose Shape

If you fall off the fitness wagon, shake the dust off, realize you're not a bad person, and climb back on. First, note what you were able to stick with on a regular basis, and be sure to include this in your next go-round. Then try to pinpoint what triggered your slip-up. Was it a change in your schedule? The weather? An injury? Boredom? Fatigue? Unsupportive friends or family members? Lack of motivation? (Hint: If your stationary bike has become the place you hang clothes to drip-dry, home may not be the place you find motivation.)

Congratulate yourself on the progress you made, rather than lamenting where you fell short. For example, if you wanted to drop 25 pounds and shed 15, don't despair— celebrate how far you progressed!

Don't be afraid to ask a pro to help you overcome stumbling blocks. If you can't seem to stick with your fitness program, for example, sign up for a couple of sessions with a personal trainer. If eating right keeps going all wrong, ask a dietitian, a nutritionist, or a personal chef for help.

now what do I do?

Answers to common questions

Q I can barely get my little ones to eat anything other than hot dogs with ketchup. They're never going to go for this healthy-eating business. Any suggestions?

Sure. After all, these are the same kids who ate mashed green bean goop in a jar without protest as babies. The same goes now: As the parent, you decide which foods to offer and when and where to serve them. Leave it to your kids to decide what and how much to eat.

When kids know that what's on the table is what's for dinner, they will eat if they are hungry—but if their eating is already going to the dogs, it might take some work to get you back to when they scarfed down vegetables. At your family meeting, explain to your little ones that when dinner is served they should take at least one bite of each offering on their plate, as there won't be anything else served later. If they don't like what they try, they don't have to eat it. (Try to include one healthful item you know they'll eat.) If they choose not to eat, the consequence will be that they're hungry.

To make healthful eating fun, ask them to help you choose interesting fruits or vegetables at the store, or to help you plant and pick fruits or vegetables in the garden. Encourage them to help cook, as most kids love to sample something they've prepared. Never mind if they make a mess or aren't exacting with the measurements. Stick to your resolve, and be patient and upbeat. Don't make food a battleground or use it as a punishment or a reward.

Q I never know whether I should exercise when I'm sick. Any suggestions?

Studies show your body can manage a good workout in spite of a runny nose or a little congestion. But if your cold is accompanied by fever, fatigue, vomiting, a deep cough, an infection, or muscle or joint aches—all of which stress your body—take a few days off and let your body heal. If you're unsure, check with your doctor.

Q I exercise, but I still feel stressed out. What can I do?

A key component of fitness—relaxation—is often overlooked. Spend a few minutes each day shaping up your psyche in addition to your body. Shift your focus inward and try to clear your head of all the day's noise. Then try to relax yourself from toe to head, focus on your breathing, and visualize yourself as fit, content, and peaceful. Don't let your to-do list take time away from your sleep. Sleep deprivation can trigger weight gain, stress, and—as you try to replenish your energy supply—overeating.

HELPFUL RESOURCES

BOOKS
Fitness Walking for Dummies,
Liz Neporent
Strategies for getting fit through walking.

Workouts for Working People,
Mark Allen with Bob Babbitt and Julie Moss
Helps you find time to work out, offers tips on aerobics, strength-training, stretching, and working out with a partner.

Quick and Healthy Cooking for Dummies, Tim Turner and Lynn F. Fischer
More than 150 recipes for healthful dishes that you can make in less time than it takes to watch a sitcom. Also includes time-saving cooking tips.

MAGAZINES
Cooking Light
800-336-0125
Features lots of menu ideas, recipes, recipe makeovers, advice, cooking tips, and techniques. The Web site (**www.cookinglight.com**) includes an index of all recipes that have appeared in the magazine. Search feature allows you to retrieve many of them.

index

boredom, avoiding, 177, 182
bread, 73
breaststroke, 174
breathing, 142
buddy system, 20, 84
butter substitutes, 78
buttocks, 152–153

c

caffeine, 96
calcium, 42, 52, 64
calories, 28–29
  counting, 102
  determining required

number of, 29
exercise's burning of, 107
fat intake and, 31
on food labels, 48
minimum requirements of, 88
muscle use of, 133
weight loss and, 88–89
calves
  strength training for, 151
  stretching, 119
cancer, 13, 70
carbohydrates, 34–35
  calories in, 28
  complex, 34–35
  recommended intake of, 61
  simple, 34
  in snacks, 77
cardiorespiratory fitness,
   12–13, 108
carotenoids, 47
cellulite, 102
chest
  strength training for, 14
  stretching, 117
children
  exercising with, 185–186
  healthy eating for,
   186–187, 198
Chinese food, 190
cholesterol
  controlling intake of, 31
  eggs and, 65
  exercise and, 106
  fiber and, 36
  fitness and, 13
  HDL, 31
  LDL, 31-32, 36
  shopping and, 78
  soy and, 32
chromium, 43

circuit-training, 177
clumsiness, exercise classes
  and, 128
coffee, 67
community centers, 125
cooking, healthful, 74–75, 78, 91
Cooking Light, 199
cooling down, 112–113,
  for aerobics, 176
  in strength training, 143
  stretching in and, 115
copper, 44
cross-country ski machines, 169
cross-training, 177, 182
cruciferous vegetables, 46, 70
crunches, 148

d

dairy foods, 33, 64, 72
dehydration, 113, 194
deli food, 191
deltoids (delts), 15, 144–145
desserts, 189
Dexatrim, 96
diabetes, 13
diaries. *See* notebooks
Dietary Reference Intakes
  (DRIs), 27
  of minerals, 42–45
  of vitamins, 39–41
diet drinks and pills, 96–97
diet fads, 58
  evaluating, 93–95
  high-fiber, low-fat diets, 95
  high-protein, low-carbohydrate diets, 94–95
  problems with, 92–93
dietitians, 69, 84, 197
diets. *See* weight, managing
dining out, 188–191

THE AUTHORS: UP CLOSE

Carol Leonetti Dannhauser is a journalist whose work has appeared in *The New York Times, American Health, Natural Health,* and many other publications. She is a National Health Information Award winner and has had two Emmy nominations. She holds a master's degree in journalism from Columbia University.

Sandra Michaelson Warren, a freelance writer and editor, is a graduate of Tufts University and holds a master's degree in public health from Yale University. She thanks Nancy A. Held, M.S., R.D., for her nutrition advice; and Alan Mikesky, Ph.D., Associate Professor at Indiana University-Purdue University Indianapolis for sharing his expertise in exercise physiology.

Barbara J. Morgan Publisher, Silver Lining Books

Barnes & Noble Basics™
Barb Chintz Editorial Director
Leonard Vigliarolo Design Director

Barnes & Noble Basics™ *Getting in Shape*
Andrea Rotondo Editor
karen j Graphic Design
Dana Cooper Illustration
Emily Seese Editorial Assistant
Della R. Mancuso Production Manager

Picture Credits

Artville 28, 56, 82; **Comstock** 1, 5 *bottom*, 113, 120, 122, 137, 161 *top*, 164, 165, 166, 173, 186, 191 *bottom*; **Corbis** 5 *top*, 19, 30, 33, 35, 37, 39, 40, 41, 42, 43, 44, 58, 62, 64, 65, 66, 70, 74, 75, 76, 87, 88, 90, 134, 136, 138, 161 *bottom*, 169, 174, 184, 188, 190 *top*; **Eyewire** 14, 68, 96, 190 *center*; **Anne Marie Weber/FPG Int'l** 196; **PhotoDisc** 4, 9, 15, 21, 26, 45, 46, 48, 61, 85, 91, 93, 98, 101, 109, 114, 125, 141, 171, 177, 182, 190 *bottom*, 191 *top*, 195; **Rubberball Productions** 16, 106, 110, 126, 132, 155, 163; **Chuck Savage/The Stock Market** 192